7 Daily Core Exercises for Seniors

A Free and Easy Approach to Firming Your Body Within 30 Days;

Includes Routines for Sitting, Standing and Lying Down

By

Sarah Ranson

7 Daily Core Exercises for Seniors

A Free and Easy approach to Firming your Body within 30 Days;

Includes Routines for Sitting, Standing and Lying down

Contents

Introduction

We're not growing older—we're growing up. As we get to those wonderful fifties, sixties, and beyond, it's time to face this phase of life with open arms. Gone are the days of following the newest fashion diets or the craziest workout programs that make us tired. Now, we can do things at our own pace and concentrate on the most important matters—keeping our bodies strong, mobile, and feeling great from the inside out.

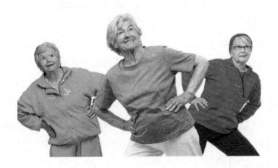

Fig. ii

That's precisely what I talk about in this book. There are no tricks or magic remedies, just a plain, lasting way of making your core strong so you can continue doing the things you love for a long time. After all, the core is the base of so much in life—better posture, more energy, fewer aches and pains. It's the key to aging well and staying youthful. This approach helps you turn flab into tone (FIT).

I'm sure you're now asking yourself -"Why exercise? At my age? No, I'd prefer a good book and cup of tea. " Believe me, I know what you're talking about. Being a senior, the last thing I want is to spend hours groaning in the gym or following an overly cheerful fitness instructor on TV. Having been through all the exercise fads under the sun in my younger days, it's demoralizing to go through the complicated routines that look like they're meant for the Olympic athletes.

But these core exercises? They're different. They're fast, easy, and fun! This special book for people over 50/60 consists of seven basic moves that will make you stronger and able to move more easily and confidently. No fancy equipment needed. Just make do with what you've got. There's no need to jump around or risk throwing your back out. Only you, a mat or a towel if you want some cushion, and maybe some light weights if you feel extra spunky.

Besides, you can do these core exercises almost anywhere - from your living room to the backyard and even your bedroom if you want to combine them with something else. A few minutes each day is all it takes to see the benefits of a stronger and leaner waist. And I tell you, there is nothing like the feeling of finally being able to bend over and tie your shoes or pick up your grandkids without having to groan out loud from the pain. It's the freedom and the ease of movement that you should have as you move through this wonderful stage of life.

I can already hear you—"But Sarah, I've got bad knees/a bum shoulder/a fussy lower back. How can I exercise?" Don't worry, my friend. These activities are both adaptable and adjustable. You can change any part that you want to fit your requirements. Keep reading to discover all the tips and tricks to make sure you're exercising safely and comfortably.

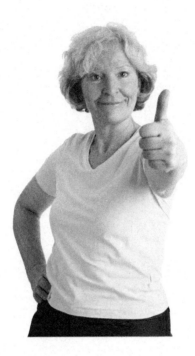

Fig. ii

"This all sounds good, but I just don't have the motivation or the discipline to keep up with an exercise routine," - I've got you covered there, too. We'll go through these core exercises together, and I'll reveal my secrets to make fitness more fun and a delightful daily routine. I'll reveal goal-setting strategies and the creative ways to sneak in the extra movement throughout your day. You'll be amazed by how these small, consistent habits can add up to big changes in just weeks.

We'll laugh together, cheer for the small achievements, and even leave with a slightly firmer backside as a gift (you're welcome!). However, the most significant outcome will be that we'll honor our bodies, raise our confidence, and build a feeling of wellness that goes far beyond the physical.

What do you think? Is your mind all set for this exciting and rewarding adventure on the way to a more stable core and a more powerful self? Let me tell you, a few days from now, this consistent effort will help you achieve FIT. You'll ask yourself why you didn't start earlier. Go for it, my friend! The future is still bright, and your best days are ahead of you.

Recommendation on How to Use This Book

I specifically designed this book to guide seniors through a series of core exercises designed to improve strength, stability, and overall fitness. To maximize the benefits, I recommend that you first read through the entire book to understand the exercises, their benefits, and the science behind them. Once you've got a good grasp of the material, you can start incorporating the exercises into your daily routine.

Suggested Approach Based on Chapter Preferences

a. *For Those Who Choose to Do the Exercises in Chapter 5 for One Month:*

Chapter 5 focuses on exercises that you can do lying down, perfect for those who prefer low-impact movements that reduce stress on the joints. These exercises are:

1. Basic Crunch

2. Leg Drops

3. Pelvic Tilts

4. Bicycle Crunches

5. Windshield Wipers

6. Marching Bridge

7. Double-leg Abdominal Press

b. *For Those Who Choose to Do the Exercises in Chapter 6 for One Month:*

Chapter 6 includes exercises that you can perform while sitting, ideal for those who might have difficulty standing for long periods. These exercises are:

1. Seated Marches

2. Seated Torso Twists

3. Seated Leg Extensions

4. Seated Side Bends

5. Seated Forward Bends

6. Seated Russian Twists

7. Seated Crunches

c. *For Those Who Choose to Do the Exercises in Chapter 7 for One Month:*

Chapter 7 contains exercises that you do while standing. They can help improve balance and stability. These exercises are:

1. Standing Side Bends

2. Hip Circle Exercise

3. Standing Torso Twist

4. Knee Lifts

5. Standing Elbow to Knee

6. Side Leg Lifts

7. Standing Plank

d. *For Those Who Choose a Mixture of the Exercises:*

For those who prefer a varied routine, combining exercises from Chapters 5, 6, and 7 can provide a comprehensive workout. Here is a suggested one-week schedule that you can repeat weekly:

Weekly Exercise Routine:

Day 1:

- Basic Crunch (Chapter 5: Back Exercises) - 3 sets of 10 repetitions

- Seated Marches (Chapter 6: Chair Exercises) - 3 sets of 10 repetitions

- Standing Side Bends (Chapter 7: Standing Exercises) - 3 sets of 10 repetitions

- Leg Drops (Chapter 5: Back Exercises) - 3 sets of 10 repetitions

- Seated Torso Twists (Chapter 6: Chair Exercises) - 3 sets of 10 repetitions

- Hip Circle Exercise (Chapter 7: Standing Exercises) - 3 sets of 10 repetitions

- Bicycle Crunches (Chapter 5: Back Exercises) - 3 sets of 10 repetitions

Day 2:

- Seated Leg Extensions (Chapter 6: Chair Exercises) - 3 sets of 10 repetitions

- Standing Torso Twist (Chapter 7: Standing Exercises) - 3 sets of 10 repetitions

- Pelvic Tilts (Chapter 5: Back Exercises) - 3 sets of 10 repetitions

- Seated Side Bends (Chapter 6: Chair Exercises) - 3 sets of 10 repetitions

- Knee Lifts (Chapter 7: Standing Exercises) - 3 sets of 10 repetitions

- Windshield Wipers (Chapter 5: Back Exercises) - 3 sets of 10 repetitions

- Seated Forward Bends (Chapter 6: Chair Exercises) - 3 sets of 10 repetitions

Day 3:

- Standing Elbow to Knee (Chapter 7: Standing Exercises) - 3 sets of 10 repetitions

- Marching Bridge (Chapter 5: Back Exercises) - 3 sets of 10 repetitions

- Seated Russian Twists (Chapter 6: Chair Exercises) - 3 sets of 10 repetitions

- Side Leg Lifts (Chapter 7: Standing Exercises) - 3 sets of 10 repetitions

- Double-leg Abdominal Press (Chapter 5: Back Exercises) - 3 sets of 10 repetitions

- Seated Crunches (Chapter 6: Chair Exercises) - 3 sets of 10 repetitions

- Standing Plank (Chapter 7: Standing Exercises) - Hold for 20 seconds, 3 repetitions

Day 4:

- Repeat Day 1 exercises

Day 5:

- Repeat Day 2 exercises

Day 6:

- Repeat Day 3 exercises

Day 7:

- Repeat Day 3 exercises

This weekly exercise routine provides a balanced and comprehensive approach to core strengthening, targeting various muscle groups through lying, sitting, and standing exercises. By repeating this plan continuously, you'll continue to build and maintain core strength, leading to improved stability, posture, and overall fitness. Remember to warm up before starting and cool down after each session as outlined in Chapters 4 and 8.

Chapter One

Starting Strong: Embracing the Journey to a Vibrant Core

Well, well, well. . . who is this? You're finally here! You deserve a pat on the back because getting this book means you've already taken the first step to a better, more vibrant you. There is no better time than now to take care of your health and life and there is no better time to achieve FIT.

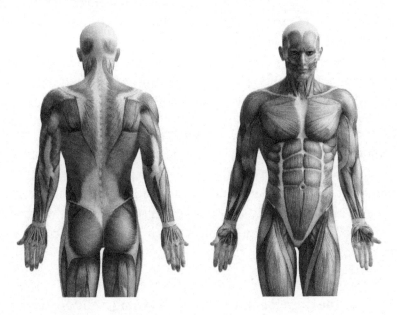

Fig. 1.1

You've managed to get here by looking after everyone else - your children, spouse, and job. However, there comes a time when we need to press that metaphoric pause button and ask ourselves, "What about me? When do I get to be the priority for a change?" The answer is today, my friend. Now, you're making a promise to yourself to take care of your body's core strength because a strong core is the gift that keeps giving.

The Significance of Core Strength as We Grow Older

The core is said to be the basis of all movement, and as we get older, having a strong and stable core becomes even more important. Reflect on it - how often have you bent over to pick something up and felt that familiar pain in your lower back? Or you may have found it hard to get up from a chair without using your arms to support you. A weak core is why so many day-to-day aches, pains, and mobility issues start to develop as the years go by.

However, what if we decided to be proactive instead of giving up and accepting a life of creaky joints and often wincing? What if we could strengthen that midsection with only a few minutes of focused core exercises every day, making our movements easier, our balance and stability better, and the groaning every time we've got to get down on the floor to play with the grandkids, a thing of the past?

Guess what! Core training does the trick. It's as if you were doing a major repair of your body's organic system. The core muscles—abs, back, hips, and everything in between—are like an invisible weight belt, bracing your spine and keeping you upright and steady as you go about your day. The denser this core foundation, the less you'll need to turn to the ice pack when you twist, bend, stretch, and move around.

It's not only about the physical advantages but also the reason for getting on the train for core strength. A strong, solid core, which is responsible for the basic body functions, makes you confident and feel infinitely more capable. There is a sense of power that comes with being able to load up the car, carry those heavy groceries, and just be fit. You're in control of your physical life rather than being limited by achy joints and a lack of stability.

Moreover, a good, strong core is the key to a fit, functional life, which reduces the risk of falls, injuries, and even some health problems such as arthritis in the later years. It's a gift you should give to yourself. You'll strengthen your abdominal muscles, which will in turn help to improve your posture and make you look more active. I'm sure you know what I mean!

Common Concerns and Cautions

Let's be honest—if you're a bit scared to begin a core workout routine, you're not the only one. You probably have a lot of concerns and "what ifs" spinning in your brain. What if I injured my back? What if my knees aren't strong enough to withstand the pressure? What if I'm just too old and inflexible for this?

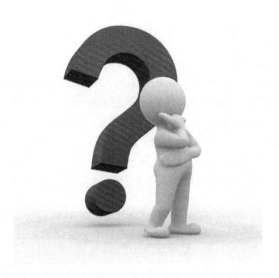

Fig. 1.2

Deep breath, my friend. I can hear those worries and am the first to tell you they're valid. After you've been struggling with chronic aches, pains, or mobility issues for years, the thought of intentionally working your core muscles can be scary. However, the most important thing to remember is that I wrote this book specifically for you. It considers your needs and limitations.

I'll never ask you to bend and pound your joints to the ground. These low-impact, joint-friendly moves help eliminate existing problems rather than worsen them. It's all about core stabilization to release pressure from sensitive areas.

Back pain is one of the most frequent causes of restricted movement as we age. You've been trying to avoid any movements that might be hard on that sensitive lower back for years, which is quite understandable. It's crucial to avoid serious injury!

Be assured that by gradually strengthening your core, you're also strengthening your body's natural back support system. The abdominal, oblique, and back muscles (I'll introduce you better to these muscles as we move on) work together to keep your spine straight and supported. That means you're much less likely to have tweaks, spasms, discomfort, and pain.

If you have short—or long-term back pain, don't worry. You'll be instructed on special modifications to make in order to safely strengthen your core and back. Some ways of modifying the exercises are simple substitutions like making some moves while sitting in a chair or not performing the exercises that cause any pain. We'll also give you useful techniques like focusing on Kinesio taping to the affected area to ease the existing back tension.

What about those who have to cope with arthritis, knee pain, or other joint problems? No problem— I've got that covered, too. You can do most of the core exercises lying down or sitting, which will eliminate any weight-bearing pressure. Also, you can use ancient medicinal practices like acupuncture and others to help control inflammation and keep your joints in good condition.

The key to the game here is to tailor the routine to your individual needs and skills. If any exercise is uncomfortable for you, you'll find the best alternative, modification, or prop to make it safe for your joints.

Other obstacles you may face are flexibility and mobility limitations. Remember, there's no reason to let these issues make you give up. You'll begin by doing the easier poses that are directed toward the minimization of gravity. Each exercise has a beginner's version, so we can start with the easy ones and then move on to the harder ones.

The Mind-Body Connection

We've already discussed all the wonderful physical advantages of having a strong, supportive core—mobility is increased, aches and pains are reduced, and balance and stability are improved. However, your body strength and fitness are only part of the battle when it comes to aging vibrantly. The mind-body connection is also significant. In other words, your mental and emotional health are just as important as physical health.

When you do your core exercises, the benefits extend beyond just achieving a strong midsection, as important as that is. You'll feel more confident and capable, and happier overall. You'll enjoy the feeling of taking control of your health through exercise and self-care.

To be specific, when you begin to exercise regularly and build up your body's core, you create a life- transforming chain reaction. You begin to feel stronger physically, which in turn makes you stronger mentally and more mentally resilient. Suddenly, you realize that you're capable and strong, and this beneficial attitude spills over into all areas of your life.

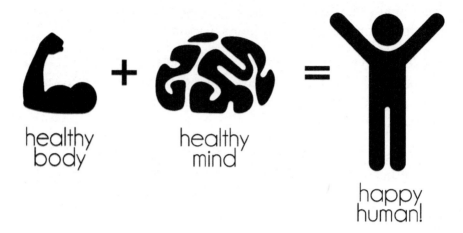

healthy body + healthy mind = happy human!

Fig. 1.3

It's as if you're finally allowing yourself to put your needs and well-being first, instead of being the last on the to-do list. I'm here to tell you that transforming your attitude in this way creates an incredible feeling of empowerment. You begin to regard your body as something to be celebrated and taken care of, not just a shell that creates problems for you as you grow old.

Each time you do the core exercise, you prove to yourself that you can care for your whole body, mind, and spirit. You're building a positive circle of self-encouragement and motivation to drive you further.

Plus, remember the mood-lifting effect of exercise! We all know that the endorphin rush you get after a great workout. Strengthening exercises, including the ones in this book, can help you reduce anxiety, depression, and the symptoms of chronic stress. By concentrating on rhythmic breathing and conscious use of the core muscles, you're starting the natural process of body relaxation.

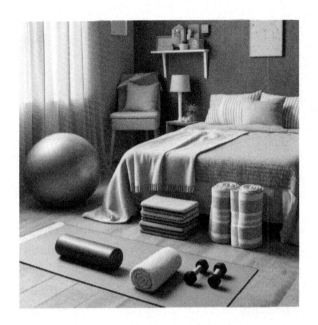

Fig. 1.4

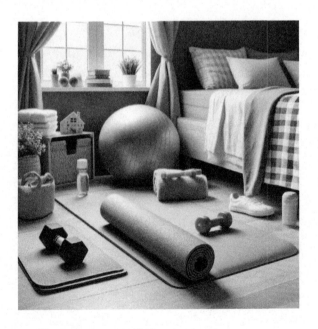

Fig. 1.5

This mind-body connection is a two-way street. When you train your physical core, you become more focused, present, and calm.

Getting Started: Creating the Conditions for Success (Fig. 1.4 and 1.5)

You're now at the starting line. I know that you're excited to start strengthening your core. However, before we begin, I need to make sure that you have the right environment for the exercises.

In fact, the right exercise setup can be the deciding factor when it comes to whether or not you'll have a good time. Maybe you're thinking you could just lie on the living room floor and start crunching. But where is the joy in that? You should make building an atmosphere that lets you enjoy your daily routine part of the core training process. We want to create an atmosphere of comfort, support, and the feeling of "Heck yeah, let's do this thing!"

Start getting to know the space where you plan to exercise. In your best scenario, you'll have a specific place for doing core work, even if it's just a cozy corner of the bedroom or a cleaned-off space in the basement. Take some time setting up your area so that it's your personal care island!

You could put down a yoga mat, towel, or exercise pad to protect those joints. Also, don't overlook the props you might need, such as a stability ball, dumbbells if you want to make it harder, or a thick book or rolled towel to modify the exercises. Having all your gear in one place makes you less likely to skip sessions.

So let the fun begin.

Chapter Two

Core Exercise Everyday Routine
– A Journey to Consistency

Timing Your Core Exercises

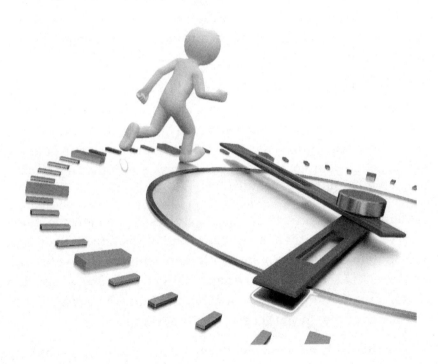

Fig. 2.1

Okay, now that we're all excited to achieve FIT and make this a regular habit, let's discuss the details. Namely, which is the best time to have your core exercise session each day? Besides, the key factor in creating a new habit is making it part of your daily life. After a while, it will feel easy and natural.

Research has proven that doing core exercises designed for a specific area in the morning, right after you've woken up fully, can be a great way to boost your energy and improve your breathing all day.

It's so refreshing to begin your day by moving intentionally and connecting with your body's powerhouse. You'll probably feel a sudden surge of alertness, and your posture will straighten up as soon as you start working on those abdominal muscles. Just be careful not to overdo the exercises on a completely empty stomach, or you could end up feeling tired. At the same time, however, you need to give yourself time to digest any food in your stomach before you exercise.

The next best time is the mid to late-morning, after your body has had time to digest your morning meal. Controlled core movements when you're feeling energized and ready to play have been proven to connect your mind and body, thus improving your balance skills. So, do your core work first and save your other daily tasks and routines for later.

If you don't have time to do your exercises in the morning, don't worry. You can do them at another time of the day that you find most suitable and convenient. If it's more suitable for you to work on the task in the middle of the day or the early evening, you should do so. It's important to choose a window of time that you'll stick to most of the time, so you get set in your new routine.

Remember to keep your meal schedule in mind when making plans. As I mentioned earlier, you need to let any food you've eaten digest before you start exercise. This is especially important when it comes to heavy meals. Had a big plate of lasagna? You should rest for a few hours before exercising. If you don't, you'll end up feeling tired and bloated.

In the end, the "best" time to core train is the one that suits your lifestyle and allows you to be at your best and most focused during each session. That would be a great way to start the day. If you're more of a laid-back evening muncher, I'm right there with you. Just make sure that whatever time you choose, you can make it a solid, permanent part of your daily self-care practice.

Now, let's find out how to transition this new core exercise routine into your daily schedule without having to worry about it.

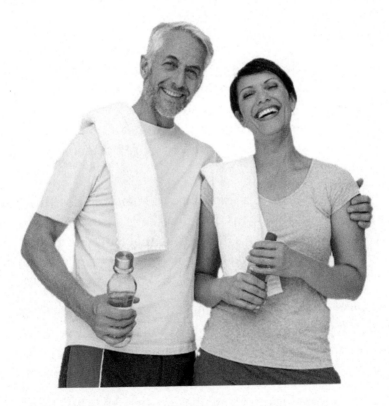

Fig. 2.2

Preparing Your Body

Okay, you've decided on what time each day you'll do your core exercise routine, and you're ready to make it a regular habit. However, before we start the moves, we should take a break and get that body ready. No, I don't mean things like squeezing into workout gear or drinking neon energy drinks. This step is about getting your muscles ready and awakening your mind-body connection using light stretching exercises.

Going in too strong too soon is the biggest guarantee of discomfort, injury, and uncontrolled frustration. Plus, it's antithetical to create an unpleasant experience when we know that your core exercises should be enjoyable. The few minutes you spend preparing and checking your breath sets the mood for a safe, pleasant, and empowering session every time.

So, let's begin with a breathing exercise. Locate a comfortable and supported sitting or lying position. Straighten your back, release the tension from your shoulders, and take a few deep breaths, and then you'll be ready to go. Observe how the air flows through your body without any hindrance. Are you more present and focused? That's step one!

We'll start from this point and lead on the inside by softly turning your spine in both directions. Imagine you're a temporary windmill that's slowly moving from side to side without any effort. This helps to relax your vertebrae, creating more room for fluid movement as we move into the core work.

Once you've attended to your spine, direct your attention to the hips and legs. Try sketching figure eights or following some circles with your feet, waking up your inner and outer thigh muscles. We'll use these guys as the key members of your main support group.

As you move your legs and feet, don't forget to keep breathing. Take a deep breath through your nose to fill your belly, then breathe out completely to relax your middle. This mindfulness breathwork is an important part of correctly using your abdominal muscles, and it helps you achieve a wonderful, centered feeling.

The last part of the warm-up is some good old-fashioned stretching! We're not talking about any deep, muscle-tearing stretches here. Instead, we'll just do a few gentle leans and extensions to enhance your mobility and circulation before we start more of a core-shaking pace.

You can sit or lie on your back, whichever is more comfortable for you. Attempt to raise your arms to the ceiling and stretch as high as possible to lengthen your whole body. Choose to pull a bit if you want to. Afterward, you should reach those arms behind you to eliminate the remaining shoulder tension. Bring your knees to your chest for a restorative hip hinge if you're on the ground.

The main goal is to create an environment where the body can move and be open without putting too much strain on it. Consider this as the preparation of the fertile soil for the core strengthening to happen. You're making and growing the moves that require more space, stability, and breath support.

As you finish the warm-up phase, take one last cycle of slow, deep breaths. This is the time to transition, set an intention for your core session, or just bask in how wonderful and ready you are.

This is the whole purpose of the warm-up process—to prepare your mind and body for each routine, to be caring and energizing instead of harsh. You've built the best jumping-off point for activating your core with control and mindfulness. Moreover, you'll find that this gives you the most out of these exercises. There will be no more straining or powering through—you'll be honoring your body's needs from the beginning to the end.

Creating a Consistent Routine

Great job on ticking all those preparation boxes! You're already demonstrating that you can go all in for this core exercise journey. However, the main question is how to convert this into a habit you'll always do.

Remember, routines are those amazing parts of life that become simpler and more fixed the more we do them. It takes a bit of effort to keep consistent with them during the first few weeks, but after that your mind and body will adjust to the new normal.

That's why I always tell my students to start small and be patient with themselves when developing a sustainable exercise routine. If you're too tough on yourself, especially from the very beginning, you'll feel overwhelmed and probably burn out and quit.

Starting small is sometimes called the "just one" method. That is, just start with focusing on getting your one core session done a day, even if it's very short. It could be as short as five minutes or as long as twenty. Just make sure you show up once a day without any special effort. Those "just ones" will accumulate most wonderfully in the long run.

A handy tip is to tie your core exercise to an existing daily habit or routine. This process is a strong psychological factor that will make your exercise routine feel like a regular part of your day.

For some people, morning may be the best time to do abs work—do a few crunches while brushing your teeth and then move to the next set as your coffee is brewing. For others, a post-lunch habit is the right one for them.

The key is to see your core exercise routine as something fun for which you've already established a habit loop rather, not a random chore that feels disruptive. You're not just finding time for it; you're turning it into a must-have part of your day that you really want to do.

Also, in the future, let's be creative with bringing extra joy and personality into your core routine. A place you love, the music you like to move to, or even a special treat you can have afterward can turn the whole process into a pleasant experience.

Have you ever had a day when you woke up and felt "blah," not even in the mood to do anything? This is where having a fully stocked fun zone around your core workout is a real game-changer. Let's be honest: When your exercise mat is next to a bowl of fresh fruit and your favorite record is already cued up to play, you're more likely to get excited and actually follow through. It's basic human psychology!

Last but not least, don't forget to make your schedule practical and changeable in case things don't go according to plan. Having a perfect, non-negotiable time to do something is good, but give yourself some room to be flexible. Your mornings are usually core-dedicated, but you can easily move that session to the evening if you oversleep or have a meeting. You're in charge here!

The aim is to develop a sustainable habit, not a limiting obligation that makes you feel guilty or resistant. Make changes where you like while making sure you stay gentle. Keep yourself accountable to be present in some way, shape, or form each day.

If you can turn this core routine into something you enjoy, that's when the real magic starts. You'll long for those movement endorphins and the increased mobility, stability, and overall excellence you get from constantly strengthening your body's core. And at that time, my friend, you're really there!

Slowing Down and Being Steady

Okay, let's all take a deep breath—in the nostrils and out the mouth. There we go. Do you know why we're doing that? Tell us that this core exercise life is a marathon, not a sprint. You don't have to jump to the finish line right at the beginning!

I'll give you an example: One of the greatest mistakes that people make when they start a new fitness program is that they go full out from the first day. They get hit by this gung-ho motivation storm, thinking that the only way to see results is through intense daily grind sessions and pushing their limits to the maximum.

Unfortunately, this is unsustainable. It's the surest way to end up with burnout and injury. . Most importantly, it misses the whole idea of what strengthening your core is all about.

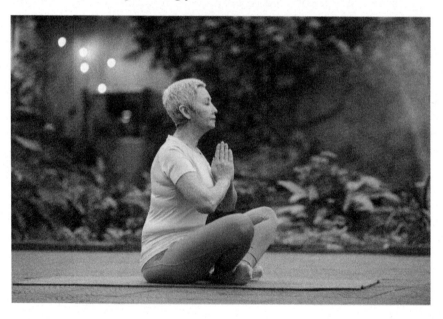

Fig. 2.3

This is not what you used to do in high school P.E. class, people. We're not trying to find out who can do the most excruciating ab routine or who can push past their physical limits. Certainly not. This practice aims to do it mindfully, pay attention to your body's capabilities and limitations, and gradually build solid core strength to make you feel empowered instead of tired.

It's a bit against the mainstream. In a world where we're always told to work more, go faster, and be relentless, the thought of taking a slower, lower-intensity life can be almost heretical at first. However, when it comes to core training for us fabulous older adults, it's the best thing to do.

This is why I ask you all to be patient and kind to yourselves as we go through the core exercises together. Ease is the key word here - easing into new movements, easing up if something doesn't feel quite right, and the mindset that building core strength is a gradual, imperfect process is what you should embrace.

Occasionally, you might hear a voice of self-doubt say, "This is too easy. I should be doing more." Just notice it, thank it for trying to be helpful, and re-commit to going at your own reasonable pace. The intensity will increase naturally if and when your body is ready. However, the outcome will be the opposite if you force it.

My intention is to create a safe, nonjudgmental environment for you to discover your body's specific abilities without any unnecessary pressure or stress. If that implies that you'll have to spend a few weeks on the beginner versions of the core exercises, so be it! It's very liberating to create that strong foundation first.

The human body is a miracle in how it reacts to changes. You'll always be doing those elementary movements, and your muscles will get used to the new tasks. Hastening or jumping ahead, to be precise, only goes against the natural biological process of learning.

So, let's change your definition of success for this revolutionary journey. Instead of measuring your progress by how fast you can do hundreds of intense crunches, you should be happy for the small victories. Things like:

- Feeling more solid, balanced, and integrated as you reach your core.

- The next poses or positions should be held a few seconds longer than the previous week.

- In fact, I look forward to your core routine as a kind of self-care.

- Realizing everyday activities like getting up from chairs or bending over seems easier.

These are the real indicators of the sustainability of your progress in terms of your core strength. Not the number of repetitions you can push yourself to do by clenching your teeth and not paying attention to the messages your body is sending.

This is true because, let's be honest, what can be more demotivating and less enjoyable than constant pain, strain, or injury? Thus, the fact that there is a buffer for care and patience guarantees that this core work will be a pleasant and empowering investment in your mobility and independence for many years to come.

Finally, that's the main point, isn't it? We're not striving for six-pack abs or fitness model bodies here. We're improving our quality of life and preventing the aches, pains, and imbalances that can occur if we don't take care of our core.

Accept the fact that your real strength is to be balanced—to know when to push yourself and when to relax and respect your body's needs. Sustainability over intensity. Listening over bullying. Turn that into your main exercise motto.

I can tell you that after thirty days of faithfulness to low-intensity core routines, you'll be amazed by how much more powerful, stable, and energetic you are—all without overdoing it or sacrificing your enjoyment of the process.

Who is up for redefining strength and enjoying the journey ahead? Nod slowly if that's you, and then let's kick-off!

Chapter Three

The ABS-olute Truth:

The Surprising Science Behind Those Core Muscles

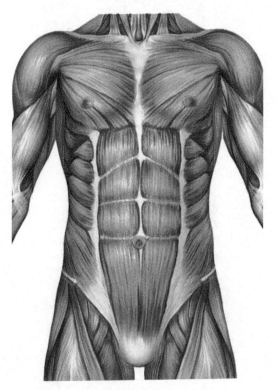

Fig. 3.1

Welcome, my friend to another wonderful adventure to the stronger, fitter you. Fasten your seatbelts because we're just about to embark on a journey that will make you the king or queen of the world!

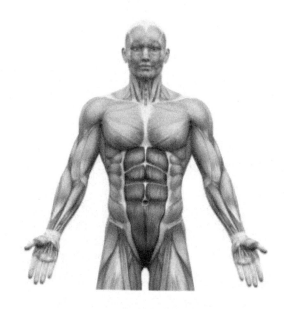

Fig. 3.2- Rectus abdominis

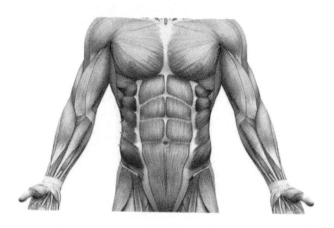

Fig. 3.3- Oblique Muscles

TRANSVERSE ABDOMINIS MUSCLE

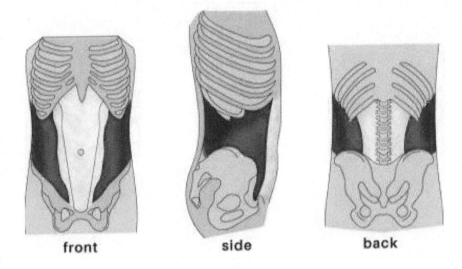

front   side   back

Fig. 3.4- Transverse Abdominis

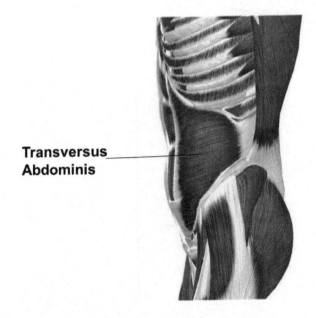

Fig. 3.5- Transverse Abdominis

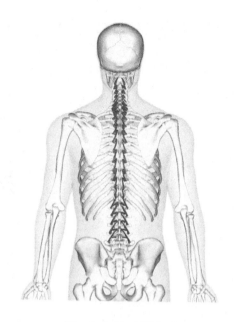

Fig. 3.6- Multifidus

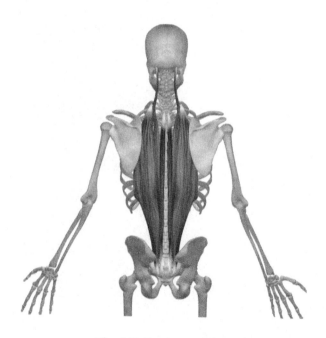

Fig. 3.7- Erector spinae

The Significance of Core Strength for Golden Oldies (Let's look at it more closely).

A. Improved mobility and physical performance

OK, it's time to face the music. The strength of the core muscles is the main thing that unlocks a new level of mobility and physical performance. Try to picture yourself being able to bend down and tie your shoes without feeling like you're participating in a contortionist's performance. Or lifting heavy groceries from the car without straining your back. You might even be so into it that you'll dance at the next family gathering (just make sure you tell the grandkids beforehand).

B. A higher degree of balance and postural stability

However, that's not all, folks! A strong core also leads to better balance and postural stability, which in turn makes us trip, slip, and fall less. You can walk those uneven sidewalks and climb those tricky steps as if you were a professional, leaving your friends and family in awe of your new grace and poise (and maybe a little bit jealous, but that's OK!).

C. The lowered probability of falls and injuries

Falls also cause fear among older people, and a weak core is a major factor in them. However, don't worry, my friends, because strengthening those core muscles will decrease your chance of falling and getting injured considerably. Picture the tranquility of mind that you get when you know that you're less likely to slip and fall and end up with a broken hip or even worse.

Now you know all about the awesome benefits of core strength for us, the older adults. Believe me, when you feel the change in your life, you'll be angry with yourself for not having started earlier.

The Principles of Core Muscles.

A. Working on the core muscle group.

Okay, now we'll start getting more into the details. I'm aware that anatomy might be perceived as a boring subject, like watching paint dry, but believe me, I'm going to make it so much fun that you'll wish your high school biology teacher was half as entertaining!

Your core is like the best friend that literally never leaves you and always supports you! This powerful team of muscles is the built-in support system for your whole body; it's the one that keeps you standing, stable, and ready to face whatever life throws at you.

If you didn't have your core, you would be as wobbly as a newborn giraffe trying to stand for the first time. Can you imagine? There you'd be, stumbling at the slightest wind, unable to reach for something on the top shelf or bend down to tie your shoes. To be honest, you might even need a spotter just to sit on the couch without falling on the cushions! Talk about a nightmare.

But don't be afraid, my friends. With a firm core, you'll be the one leaving others in awe of your grace, poise, and fabulousness. It's as if your team of superheroes is living inside you, waiting to rush in and save the day when you need them.

So, let's start with these main muscle groups and give them the love and the attention they need. After all, they've been working hard in the background all these years, keeping you upright and in good health, without any thank-you or a parade in their honor. It's about time we started to appreciate them!

B. The function of each core muscle

Next, let's introduce the star players in this core muscle team. We also have the rectus abdominis, the famous "six-pack" muscle. . These bad boys are the ripped cover models of the core world; they get all the attention and admiration.

But don't be misled by their good looks - they're more than just pretty faces. The rectus abdominis is the main muscle that flexes your spine and protects your internal organs. It's as if you have your very own built-in superhero suit that protects your valuable internal organs from harm, looking fantastic at the same time.

After that, we have the obliques, which are like your body's natural corset. These side muscles are the silent hero of core stability; they help you twist, bend, and move easily. Drop those narrow waist trainers; the obliques are the ones who really do the job of creating a perfect, sculpted, and strong middle section that's also functional.

Can you bear the thought of doing a simple thing like tying your shoes without these incredible muscles to help you? You'd be as stiff as a rusty tin soldier and unable to bend and contort your body into the necessary positions. No, thank you!

Besides, the transverse abdominis, the deep, hidden treasure that acts as a natural weight belt, supporting your spine and internal organs, should not be left out. This muscle is like the ultimate multitasker, always keeping everything in order while you're busy lifting, carrying, and being a total badass.

The transverse abdominis is like a support system for your body. Without it, you would be as helpless as a wet noodle, flopping around and putting yourself at risk of all sorts of injuries and back pain. Yikes!

But wait, there's more! The multifidus and erector spinae are the dynamic duo of back support. They'll help you maintain that upright posture we all desire. Imagine yourself being able to stand straight and proud without the need for your well-meaning (but sometimes nagging) friends and family to keep reminding you.

These are the muscles that are the real heroes of good posture. They fight the bad guys of slouching and hunching, who want to turn us all into a bunch of human question marks. With their assistance, you'll be able to keep your head held high and walk with confidence. You'll be the one people look at wherever you go.

It's as if you have your very own team of superheroes living inside you, each of them with a unique set of powers, and they work together to keep you strong, stable, and ready to face life's challenges.

Thus, there you have it – a humorous, inside view of the amazing anatomy of your core muscles. Who would have thought that the study of one's body could be this much fun? Now it's time to use these bad boys and start shaping your dream of a rock-solid midsection. Your main crew is all set and begging you to say, "Let's do it," so they can show their superpowers.

The Science Behind Core Strengthening

A. *The physiological reactions to core exercises*

OK, my friends. Let's be nerds and talk about the interesting science behind these core-blasting exercises. Let me explain just to show you that I'm not going to start talking in a language that only some people can understand. This stuff is fantastic, you know.

When you work out your core muscles, you're getting in shape, looking great (a big plus), and improving your health. You'll start a whole chain of physiological responses that will make you feel like a million dollars!

You'll give your body a full-scale tune-up, increasing the blood flow and oxygen delivery to your muscles, boosting your metabolism, and even enhancing your general physical function. Who would have thought core exercises could be that powerful?

Visualize yourself walking up a flight of stairs as if it were nothing, without feeling like you just ran a marathon. Or even just carrying those heavy grocery bags as if they were feathers, your neighbors left in awe of your superhuman strength. It's all the result of the power of core training and its amazing physiological effects.

B. Advantages of core stability training

But wait, there's more! Core stability training, which challenges your balance and core strength simultaneously, has been proven to improve performance in all kinds of activities, from sports to everyday tasks.

Suddenly, that hiking trail you've been wanting to do doesn't look so hard, and those household chores that bother you become a piece of cake. You may even start dancing at your next family party. Just let the grandkids know beforehand, so they don't spill their juice boxes in shock!

It's as if you're opening a new world of coolness, where your age and physical problems are no longer your obstacles. The whole world is at your feet with a strong, stable core, and you're the pearl shining bright and ready to face any challenge.

C. The significance of correct form and technique

I know what you're thinking: "Sarah, this is all well and good, but what if I do these exercises wrong and I end up looking like a flailing inflatable tube man outside a used car lot?" Don't be afraid, my friends! The right form and technique are the basics of a good performance, and I'm here to give you that information.

Do you recall that time your kids or grandkids tried to show off their fancy yoga poses at the family barbecue but ended up looking a bit like a tangled heap on the lawn, their limbs all over the place and hot dog buns scattered everywhere? Let's not even think of that possibility.

I'll be with you every step of the way, and I'll also make the whole thing engaging and fun, to make it more interesting. You'll be doing those core exercises like a pro in no time. And who knows, maybe your remarkable core strength and perfect posture will cause awe and envy at the next family gathering!

Chapter Four

Preparing Your Body for Success: The Warm-up Essentials

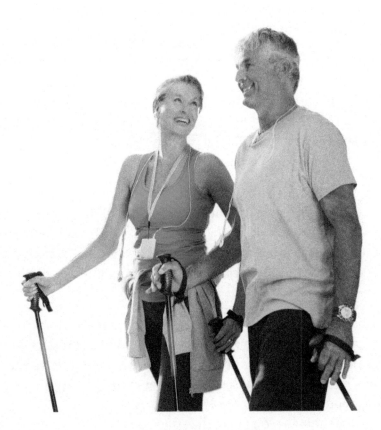

Fig. 4.1

Warm-ups are often forgotten but necessary for any exercise regimen. At first glance, you may not see much action here, but let me assure you, these simple preparations are no joke. The fact that people don't spend time stretching before core work (or any exercise) is a perfect example of when a little prevention goes a long way when it comes to potential injuries.

Some of you probably already want to pinch me and say, "But Sarah, warm-ups are so boring! I'd rather just skip it and get to the actual workout." And yes, I used to think the same way. There is no better feeling than jumping into a new routine with lots of energy and massive motivation. But you'll likely end up limping around like a bow-legged human corkscrew 10 minutes later because you skipped the warm-up.

Let me share a funny memory. On one family reunion, my boisterous cousin, Vinnie, got carried away. Instead of following the warm-up drills, he opted to do away with the stretching exercises and jumped straight into a game of basketball. Two minutes in, a big bang was heard around the yard - Vinnie suffered a hammy injury! That poor man spent the remainder of the weekend limping around with a bag of frozen peas lodged in his crotch. Not a good look.

The message of the story? Stretching is critical to ensure muscles are prepared for the tasks ahead and avoid awkward (and painful) mishaps. It's like warming up your car on a chilly winter morning before going for a fast drive on the highway. That wake-up time enables everything to wake up and get ready to go, not jolt the engine in your car.

Your body also requires the same treatment, especially as we grow older, and our muscles become more recalcitrant. A proper warm-up takes the muscles from their resting position and allows them to move smoothly. It increases blood circulation and oxygen supply throughout your body and gradually transitions your body into full gear. It will not take long to realize that your flexibility and range of motion have increased significantly after a few minutes of warm-up.

However, the advantages don't end with preventing injuries and enhancing flexibility. Contrary to popular opinion, scientific evidence indicates that warming up can enhance your exercise performance since it raises the rate of heartbeats, panting, and energy delivery to the active muscles. That means that you'll not get as tired as fast, so you can push through your core routine.

Deep Breathing Exercises

Alright, we'll begin by tapping into the powerhouse of your entire existence: your breath.

I know what you're thinking. Just breathing? Really, that's the best topic you can come up with? You might wonder, how can just breathing in and out be a workout? But let me explain. I'm about to share information that will revolutionize your basic workout routine.

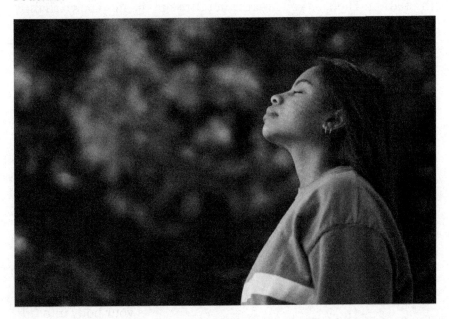

Fig. 4.2

Breath is the very life force of existence, which is why it serves as the perfect precursor to these soulful, invigorating exercises for the core region. All that we'll be doing shall be rooted in your breath and the use of the inner core muscles. Incorporating the practice of breathwork from the beginning ensures that you're grounded, alert, and optimally poised.

Now, let's start by sitting or lying down in a comfortable position. If you want, slowly blink, join your hands, and focus on the inner experience. I mean the breathing pattern as you inhale through your nostrils and exhale through your mouth or nose. Is it surface-level or profound? Steady or erratic? Just observe without judgment.

Let's try something I call 'belly buddhas.' While inhaling via your nose, imagine the air entering your lower abdomen and making your belly look like an inflating Buddha. It's also important to allow the ribs and the upper abdominal area to expand during the inhalation. Then, as you breathe out through the lips you've slightly opened, pull your belly button towards the spine, emptying all the air in your lungs.

Inhale and exhale for a few seconds each; be calm and steady as you breathe. If your mind gets distracted (as it often does), focus on the breath entering and leaving the lower abdominal area. Try to put a hand on your lower belly, as this can also help to draw attention to that area.

As you go on with these deep belly breaths, your body should start feeling heavy on the mat as you relax more and more. All pre-routine tension or fidgeting will subside, and you will be enveloped in an aura of preparedness and readiness. This is your mind-body connection working at its best!

Once you've achieved a comfortable meditation-like flow, you can expand the outer layer of your abdomen more on the inhales, almost as if there's a beach ball inside your stomach. As you breathe out, maintain the tone of those strong, deep abdominal muscles, directing your breath through your pelvic region. Observe the micromovement in your core with each cycle, but don't try to produce it independently.

Do you feel it? That wonderful sensation of your body expanding through your lungs and into your belly as you inhale? Is the sensation of any stiffness in the back or shoulders being eased and vanished? This is your pre-core routine reset, a way of preparing a positive and focused environment for the actual work to be accomplished.

Mental Preparation

Let's do some vivid visualization. Do you want to increase your vitality and be able to move around freely, so you can remain productive and live a healthy life even in your senior years? Do you want that feeling you get when you feel strong, balanced, and powerful again in your own skin? Or perhaps your goal is simpler and more practical – you need to be able to walk, run, jump, or lift without pain.

Regardless of your 'why,' remember and define it as clearly as possible and bring it to the forefront of your mind. This intention will be your compass, which will help if you lose your way or have issues. If the voice of resistance ever rises and says, "This is too hard... you're too old for this," you can always go back to your intention like a life preserver.

With that understanding in mind, let's focus on the mindset concept. At the center of this whole process (and I couldn't help but use the word 'core' here) is the message that you don't need to change, to become different, to strive for more, to seek happiness – you're already enough just as you are in this moment. You don't have to struggle, stress, twist, or contort yourself to the point where you become a pretzel. It's about being in your body with grace and love and being comfortable in it.

This warm-up period we've designed is the best time to take advantage of this laid-back attitude. As you breathed and stretched, did you catch thoughts like, "I should be able to do this by now" or "I'm too tired to do this," or maybe "I'll never be able to do that deep stretch" or "I'm so inflexible"? Those are just limitations we put into our own boxes.

Rather, I encourage you to enter each movement with the same spirit of wonder that children do. If a stretch doesn't feel good, don't try to force it – instead, step back and rediscover what feels good. If your body feels like it needs to groove and do the silly dance, then yes, shake that thing your mother gave you. This is about listening to what your body has to say about what it wants to get involved with, not about forcing your body to do something it doesn't want to do.

Well, here is some serious inspiration for you, my dear reader and friend Miriam. This 72-year-old lady's warm-up looks like something out of Cirque du Soleil. She will do deep backbends and even pretend to kick herself in the head, all while giggling about her bones and how she is entertaining the neighbors. I believe Miriam is that ageless, playful spirit in all of us, and that's why she is so relatable.

Of course, I'm not suggesting you mimic her advanced exercises, just that you try to use her enthusiasm as a reference point. Take that happy, non-critical attitude and bring it to your own warm-up. Loosen up and let yourself go with it! Perhaps include some 'jazz hands' when you're done with a fantastic stretch, or give yourself a twerking of the behind after a perfect backbend. Why the heck not? No one else is paying attention to what you're doing, which will make you feel even more alive!

The best strategy here is to be kind to the body where you find it in the present moment. So, don't think you're behind because of today's performance or try to compete with anyone else's journey of tomorrow. My Miriam might be able to kick into a Scorpion pose, but I sure as heck can't ... and that's A-OK! We're just here to appear and present ourselves as we are.

With this approach of waiting, having fun, and leaving all prejudice at the door, this whole process of core strengthening is the physical body that gains energy, the mind, and the spirit. You're flexing way more than just your muscle fibers here – you're also exercising your patience, courage, and self-esteem.

Now, that's a warm-up for the whole darn self! It prepares us for the core routines to be initiated from a place of strength instead of dogmatic strictures or negative self-talk. We're here to dance, breathe, and, most importantly, have fun while discovering the greatness of our bodies.

So, let that energy of curiosity and compassion flow through you now. Relax, release any remaining anxiety and get ready to transmute this enchanting attitude into our focus on the core muscles. We're heating up a lot more than our clothes today. We're also igniting our shining souls!

Checklist and Tips

We've learned a lot as we prepared our minds and bodies for the task of doing our core strengthening exercises like a superstar!

But first, let me stop and summarize some of the key points before we move to the core routines. There are clear and simple points to remember before every session, and this is part of your mental preparation. Once your mind is prepared, you'll be ready to start achieving core strengthening.

So, here's our warm-up rundown! Grab your pen and paper, so you can write down all these points. You might like to keep these close at hand. Maybe you could stick it on the refrigerator, or put it next to where you exercise.

The first step involves making sure your space is suitable and has the right atmosphere. Get rid of any clutter and unnecessary distractions. Think about dimming the lights or putting on some music to help get you focused. If you're going to be exercising on the floor, you should put down a washable yoga mat or a folded towel to spare your knees. Gather any necessary equipment that you may require, like blocks, massage balls, or resistance bands.

When your sacred space is prepared for the show, it's time for the first and the most important part: the warm-up! Here's how it should go:

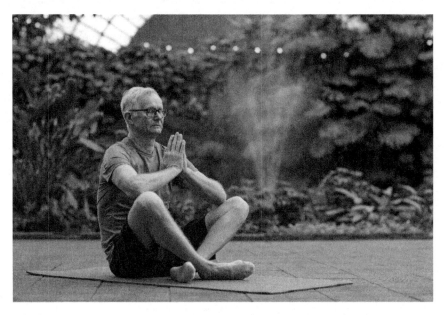

Fig. 4.3

1) Breathwork – Inhale 5 to 10 full, slow breaths with the intention of grounding. Pay more attention to the enlargement of the abdomen during inhalation, so that you engage the deep core muscles.

2) Embodiment Practice—Take two to three minutes to just be in your body through breathing. Check for tension and deliberately

let go of it in the areas where you find it. Seek clarity on why you're engaging in this practice.

3) Last Check-In – Run your hands from top to bottom over your body, feeling if you can sense any additional tension. Do we still have anything feeling restricted or needing a little more warm-up love?

Fig. 4.4

And that's it. You're now warm and ready to proceed to the core strengthening exercises, feeling comfortable and protected. You should be proud!

Of course, all of the items on this list are just recommendations—you can adjust them to your own needs and desires for the day. Perhaps some don't feel meaningful to you, or you would prefer to incorporate an additional breathwork exercise. Go for it!

The key is to create a warm-up routine that resonates with your body's energy and benefits your soul. One that forms a positive feedback loop, where you begin to look forward to winding down before charging into the main work.

Make your warm-up routine special and sacred instead of just a bunch of exercises to suffer through. Use flameless candles, music, or strings of twinkling lights to create a tranquil atmosphere. Before you start, spray yourself with a good quality body mist to make yourself feel more comfortable. Or wear your favorite shawl or slippers while you're doing your breathing exercises. The more you can transform this prep period into a special little spa day, the less chance there is that you'll skip it!

Chapter Five

Exercises on The Back

Now let's get started with the actual exercises! This chapter is tailor-made for you. Aging might bring aches in places you didn't expect, like sore knees and stiff hips, but it doesn't need to stop you from strengthening your core. Let's get started with some simple, effective exercises that you can do lying down, ensuring every step is easy to follow.

Basic Crunch

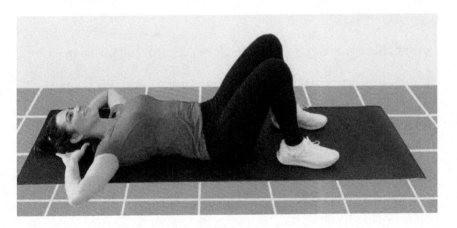

Fig. 5.1a

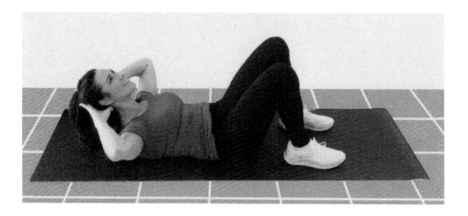

Fig. 5.2b

Setup: Lie flat on your back on a comfortable mat with your knees bent and feet flat on the floor.

Action: Place your hands behind your head lightly supporting it. Engage your core by pulling your belly button towards your spine.

Movement: Lift your shoulders off the mat slightly, keeping your lower back pressed to the floor. Hold this crunch position for a few seconds.

Return: Slowly lower yourself back to the starting position.

Repeat: Perform this movement 10-15 times.

Benefits:

A Basic Crunch is a good exercise for articulating your rectus abdominis muscles (the muscles forming your six-pack) and the obliques (muscles on the sides of your stomach). Here's what this exercise is doing for you:

1. Building Core Strength: This way, you're not merely stretching your arms; by lifting your shoulders off the mat and crunching your abdominal muscles, you're contracting and training those core

muscles. It also contributes to developing strong muscles in your stomach, which are important in supporting the spine.

2. Improving Spinal Support: Your core muscles function as your own internal girdle, supporting your backbone. When doing the Basic Crunch, activating your rectus abdominis assists in stabilizing your spine while decreasing pressure on your back muscles.

3. Enhancing Balance and Stability: To balance and not fall easily, you need strong muscles in the middle part of the body. This becomes even more important as you age. The benefit of the Basic Crunch is to build up the core muscles that are essential to keeping your balance and preventing accidents, such as falling.

4. Increasing Functional Mobility: Basic actions such as exercising, standing, sitting, walking, running, lifting, and carrying, all require core strength. As the Basic Crunch strengthens the abdominal muscles to allow for better lifting of the upper body against the lower body, doing this exercise will help make these functional movements easier and more comfortable for you.

5. Boosting Metabolic Rate: As mentioned earlier, the Basic Crunch is not considered a heavy exercise. However, it does call for the contraction of several muscles and, despite the low intensity, could help to slightly increase your Basal Metabolic Rate during and after the crunches. It can also enhance the rate at which calories are burned and, therefore, help to promote healthier weight regulation.

The Basic Crunch's main purpose is strengthening the abdominal muscles. However, the obliques, hip flexors, and lower back muscles are also worked during the exercise to a certain degree. The Basic Crunch is incredibly valuable because it engages all of your core muscles, which is why it is so effective at making your core stronger and more stable.

Be sure to perform with correct technique and posture to ensure the movements are as effective as possible and prevent injury. Ensure the lumbar region of your back remains in contact with the floor, your abdominals are switched on, and you're performing the movements in a careful, deliberate way.

Leg Drops

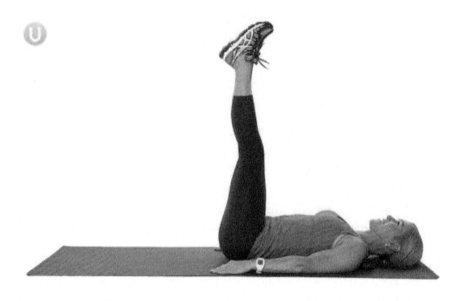

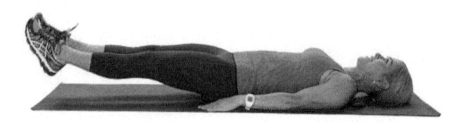

Fig. 5.3

Setup: Lie on your back with your legs raised straight up towards the ceiling, hands flat beside you for stability.

Action: Engage your core and slowly lower one leg towards the mat, keeping the other leg still and straight.

Movement: Lower the leg as far as you can while maintaining a flat lower back on the mat.

Return: Slowly raise the leg back up to the starting position.

Repeat: Alternate legs and perform 10-12 repetitions per leg.

Benefits:

The Leg Drops exercise primarily targets your lower abdominal muscles, also known as the lower rectus abdominis or the "lower abs. "Here's what this exercise is doing for you:

1. Strengthening the Lower Abs: When you bend one of the legs towards touching the mat while the other remains raised a little, you realize that the lower abdominal muscles are working. This exercise is designed to focus specifically on the area and help you develop the tone and power in your stomach area that is not worked out as often as others.

2. Improving Core Stability: As you perform the Leg Drops, you'll mostly feel the work on your lower abs, but the movement also strengthens all other stomach muscles, including your obliques and the deep inner core muscles. Unlike other yoga poses that may only focus on the core area, this activation strengthens your core foundation and better supports your body.

3. Challenging Core Control: As you lower and raise each leg, your lower back should stay flat on the mat. This requires good core strength and bilateral coordination. This exercise helps to improve the proper muscle position of the spine, which enhances your ability to have good posture throughout the day.

4. Increasing Flexibility: The Leg Drops exercise activates your hip flexors and stretches the hamstrings. It can also enhance muscle flexibility in these areas, which may help make you less prone to injury.

5. Boosting Metabolic Rate: Unlike other intense weight training exercises, Leg Drops can help to boost your metabolic rate. They give several muscle groups, such as your core, hip flexors, and hamstrings, a solid workout. As Leg Drops can help improve your metabolic rate during and after the exercise, they can be useful for weight loss over the longer term.

This exercise is particularly effective in place of crunches. Still, it must be performed correctly to ensure that you don't place too much pressure on the vertebrate in your lower back. It is also important to keep your abdominals engaged throughout this exercise, while ensuring that your lower back remains flat on the mat as you slowly and carefully perform the movements. Also, the spine must be kept at a neutral curvature, being conscious not to adopt the habit of an arch or rounded back.

Remember, Leg Drops mainly work the lower ab muscles, which can be quite tricky to exercise rigorously. This exercise may be done as a standalone form of exercise or included in a larger workout. As well as firming and toning the involved muscles, doing Leg Drops should also help strengthen your abdominal region.

Pelvic Tilts

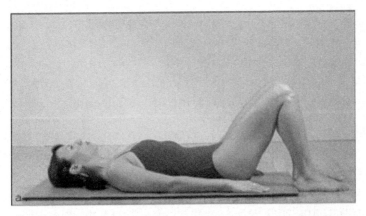

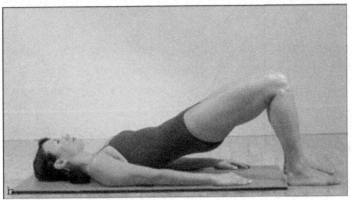

Fig. 5.4

Setup: Lie on your back with your knees bent and feet flat on the floor.

Action: Flatten your lower back against the mat by contracting your abdominal muscles and tilting your pelvis upward.

Hold: Maintain this tilted position for a few seconds.

Return: Slowly return to the starting position.

Repeat: Do this 15-20 times.

Benefits:

This exercise is called a Pelvic Tilt. It helps work out the abdominal and lower back muscles rather mildly yet effectively. It's a core stabilizing exercise and targets the deep core muscles that are crucial for good posture and spinal support. Here are the benefits you can expect from incorporating Pelvic Tilts into your routine:

1. Improved Core Stability: By drawing your belly button back and up towards your spine while flattening your stomach muscles, you directly stimulate the transverse abdominis, the most internal of your abdominal muscles. It performs the function of a fashionable tight waistband that keeps your spine stable, and your lower back strengthened.

2. Better Posture and Spinal Alignment: When you tilt during the movement, you're learning the best position to have a flat lower back on the mat, hence achieving a neutral spine. This may help make it easier for you to maintain good posture. Also, it may make you less likely to end up with the lower back aches so common in older people.

3. Increased Abdominal Strength: Although the Pelvic Tilt movement looks quite simple, this exercise involves tightening the abdominal muscles. It includes a contraction used in isometric exercise that can help you strengthen various parts of the abdominal muscle.

4. Enhanced Body Awareness: First, you concentrate some attention on the movements of the pelvic area and the tensions in your core muscles. In this way, you regain more substantial control over your positioning and muscular contractions. This would also help in other exercises and regular activities by improving form or better controlling one's own body.

5. Low-Impact Nature: It is a low-impact exercise, and therefore, seniors and people restricted by joint pain or mobility problems

can comfortably participate. As an exercise you do on the floor, it doesn't put the pressure on your joints that a higher impact, standing exercise would.

Make sure you take normal breaths when you're doing Pelvic Tilts. It's important that you avoid holding your breath, as that creates intra-abdominal pressure, including unwanted pressure on the muscles of the core area. Begin your number of Pelvic Tilt repetitions at a level that is easily manageable, then gradually increase as your body adapts.

Bicycle Crunches

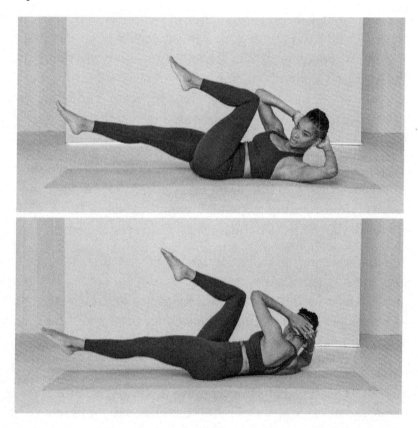

Fig. 5.5

Setup: Lie on your back with your hands behind your head and legs raised to form a 90-degree angle at your hips.

Action: Bring your right elbow towards your left knee while straightening your right leg.

Movement: Switch sides, bringing your left elbow towards your right knee while extending your left leg.

Repeat: Continue alternating sides in a 'pedaling' motion for 20-30 seconds.

Benefits:

Bicycle Crunches target your oblique muscles (located on the sides of your tummy) and rectus abdominis muscles (those ribbons you see at the front of your stomach that people often call the six-pack muscles). This dynamic exercise targets the abdominal muscles while simultaneously involving the hip flexor and lower back muscles. It's a full ab workout. Here are the benefits you can expect from incorporating Bicycle Crunches into your routine:

1. Oblique Muscle Strengthening: When applying pressure on the handle with the right hand and bringing the elbow near the left knee, you're certainly engaging the oblique muscles. This exercise's twisting action helps to build muscle endurance and strength.

2. Rectus Abdominis Activation: When you do Bicycle Crunches, the crunching motion directly compresses your rectus abdominis muscles, the ones that can create a six-pack look. You'll strengthen these muscles, which will help boost your total body stability, as well as your capacity to handle routine tasks.

3. Improved Flexibility: The pedaling leg movements in the Bicycle Crunches exercise help improve the flexibility within your hip flexors and hamstrings. Doing this exercise daily should also help with muscles such as the upper back, hip flexors, calves, anterior

tibialis, and others. You'll enhance the flexibility of these muscles, potentially giving you better mobility.

4. Increased Cardiovascular Endurance: Although not intensive, the continued coordinated motion and leg movement during Bicycle Crunches may raise your heart rate, offering you some cardiovascular exercise.

5. Core Stabilization: As with any abdominal exercise, Bicycle Crunches effectively work out all of your outer abdominal muscles, but they also use the deep core muscles like the transverse abdominis and the multifidus muscles. These muscles work together to help support the stability and correct position of the spine.

Bicycle crunches involve rotating the trunk, so it is necessary to ensure you maintain correct form, so you get the most out of this exercise, while minimizing strain on the neck. Finally, don't pull yourself up with your hands; keep your tongue behind your lower lip and your chin down. Also, move gently, especially your arms and legs. Don't make quick movements that negatively influence the position.

Windshield Wipers

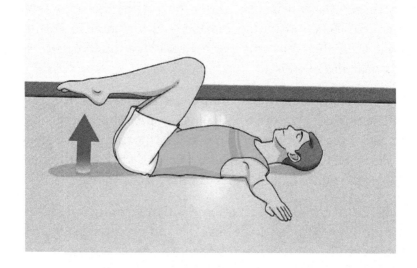

Fig. 5.6a

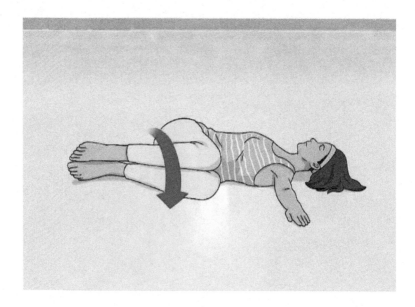

Fig. 5.6b

Setup: Lie on your back with your arms stretched out to the sides for support, legs lifted, and knees bent at 90 degrees.

Action: Rotate your legs to one side, keeping your shoulders on the floor.

Hold: Pause briefly when your legs are about 6 inches off the floor.

Return: Bring your legs back to the center and then rotate to the opposite side.

Repeat: Alternate sides for 10-12 repetitions per side.

Benefits:

The Windshield Wiper is a core exercise that works your oblique muscles, lower abdominal muscles, and hip flexors. This exercise is quite challenging physically, helping to tone your stomach and enhance your flexibility and stability. Here are the benefits you can expect from incorporating Windshield Wipers into your routine:

1. Oblique Muscle Strengthening: When moving your legs from side to side, your speed, as well as tension in your muscles, increases, and this helps strengthen your oblique muscles. These muscles provide the muscular base for rotational activities and stability, which is essential in your postural support and day-to-day activities.

2. Lower Abdominal Activation: The Windshield Wipers exercise perfectly tones your lower abdominal muscles, also commonly known as the lower rectus abdominis or lower abs.

3. Improved Flexibility: When performing this exercise, the side-to-side motion of your legs means that you need the hip flexors and the muscles in the inner thighs to have some freedom of movement. These areas that act as different facets of the windscreen wiper may be eased through regular practice, allowing you to develop better flexibility.

4. Core Stabilization: In addition to the obliques and lower abs, Windshield Wipers also work your true or inner core muscles, the transverse abdominis, and the multifidus deep muscles. These muscles assist in stabilizing the spine and allowing you to maintain correct posture.

5. Improved Balance and Coordination: When you do Windshield Wipers, you use your leg muscles to rotate your legs, while your shoulders remain flat on the floor. This helps give you the focus and stability needed. Doing Windshield Wipers will help to improve your stability in everyday life.

Make sure you use the following guidance to achieve the proper technique when doing Windshield Wipers, so you don't harm the spinal erectors. Squeeze your belly button inward as you breathe out to perform the task, and don't bend your lower back out of shape or create rounded curves in your back. Make sure that you avoid sudden or quick movements as much as possible.

Marching Bridge

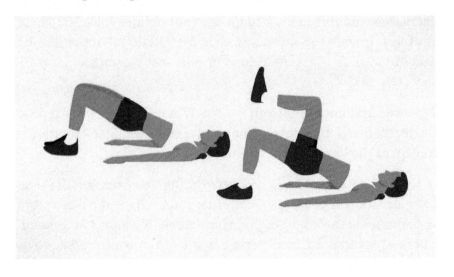

Fig. 5.7

Setup: Lie on your back with your knees bent and feet flat on the floor, arms by your sides.

Action: Lift your hips off the floor to enter a bridge position, creating a straight line from your knees to your shoulders.

Movement: While keeping your hips raised, slowly march in place by lifting one knee toward your chest, then setting the foot back down. Repeat with the other knee.

Hold: Try to maintain the bridge position steady and your hips level throughout the marching.

Return: After completing the marches on both sides, lower your hips back down to the floor.

Repeat: Perform 8-10 marches per leg, alternating legs

Benefits:

The Marching Bridge exercise is a unique and practically valuable full-core workout that impacts your abdomen, hip flexor, and gluteal muscles. Besides working on the muscles in your tummy, this exercise has the added advantage of working on your stability and balance. Here are the benefits you can expect from incorporating Marching Bridge into your routine:

1. Core Muscle Activation: By maintaining the bridge position with a ground-up posture and hips lifted off the floor, the specific muscles that are involved are rectus abdominis, which are also referred to as the "six-pack" muscles, obliques, and TVA. This constant pull assists in developing the quad muscles and provides an efficient workout for the stomach muscles.

2. Hip Flexor Strengthening: In this exercise, you must do a marching motion with your legs. It involves lifting the knees towards the chest, which targets the hip flexors. This will help to alleviate tight hip flexors. If you have this issue and experience

problems with day-to-day activities such as climbing stairs, getting out of the chair, and walking posture, the Marching Bridge may help you.

3. Glute Activation: While in the bridge position, the gluteal muscles play a crucial role in maintaining the position of the pelvis and hip joint stability. This exercise may make a great glute toning and strengthening workout, as these muscles play a major role in supporting your balance, stability, and posture.

4. Improved Balance and Coordination: Swapping leg movements while trying to balance in the middle of a bridge position is quite tricky, and will help develop your stability. It should help you improve your body awareness, balance, and coordination, hopefully improving your mobility and reducing the risk of falling.

5. Low-Impact Nature: Marching Bridge is another easy exercise that is perfect for most people who have issues with their joints or other body parts that don't allow them to exert much impact. As it is an abdominal exercise, it's best to do it when the lower back and joints are least under strain. This exercise accommodates that, as you're lying on the floor.

When you're doing the Marching Bridge, it's crucial to make the movements correctly. That way, you get maximum benefits while avoiding serious harm to the lower back. Squeeze your belly button and keep your stomach muscles tight, especially when you pull the weights towards your chest. Don't arch your lower back. Also, ensure control and smooth movement, and don't make sudden jerky actions that may affect your stance.

Double-Leg Abdominal Press

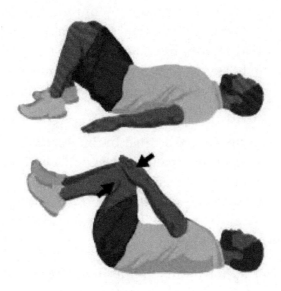

Fig. 5.8

Setup:

Lie on your back with your knees bent. Keep your back in a neutral position, not arched and not pressed into the floor. Avoid tilting your hips. Tighten the abdominal muscles.

Action: Raise your legs off the floor, one at a time, so that your knees and hips are bent at 90-degree angles. Rest your hands on top of your knees.

Movement: Push your hands against your knees while using the abdominal muscles to pull your knees toward your hands. Keep your arms straight. Hold for three deep breaths.

Return: Return to the start position and repeat.

Repeat: Perform this exercise for the desired number of repetitions, maintaining proper form throughout.

Benefits:

This exercise involves the rectus abdominis and the oblique muscles. The Double-Leg Abdominal Press exercise concentrates on the abdominal region, hips, and lower back, making it an efficient routine to exercise your abdominal muscles. Here are the benefits you can expect from incorporating the Double-Leg Abdominal Press into your routine:

1. Rectus Abdominis Strengthening: In this position—where your lower legs gently touch your palms as you pull your knees towards your hands and brace your abdominal muscles—you're flexing your rectus abdominis muscles. These muscles give the admired aesthetic display of the 'six-pack' and, when worked on, would enhance your torsos rigidity.

2. Oblique Muscle Activation: While the primary target is the rectus abdominis, this exercise also develops the oblique muscles (located on the sides of the lower abdomen). These muscles have a high level of functionality in rotational movements and stability of the trunk, making them vital in moving around and maintaining proper posture.

3. Improved Breathing Mechanics: If you contract your abdomens while performing the exercise and take deep breaths during the contraction phase, you're conditioning your diaphragm and learning correct breathing mechanics. It is noteworthy that working with different kinds of breathing can help improve the stability and functionality of the muscles. It is important to mention that all kinds of breathing can be helpful for the outer core muscles and their stability and function.

4. Hip Flexor Strengthening: This exercise will work your hip flexor muscles since one leg is lifted while the other is in contact with the ground and positioned right in front of the chest. Hip flexor muscles are a bit like pillars. You need them to be strong so you can climb stairs, rise from a chair, and even just stand erect.

5. Low-Impact Nature: The Double-Leg Abdominal Press is a low-impact exercise, so it is safe and comfortable for most people who have problems with their knees or back, or anyone who needs to avoid high-impact exercises. As you do this exercise lying down on the floor, you avoid creating pressure or pain for your joints.

6. Body Posture: It's important to maintain proper form and posture when doing the Double-Leg Abdominal Press, so that you avoid extra pressure and strain on the body's lower back region. Maintain good abdominal support, and don't bend the spine and round the lower back during the lifts. Also, try to move steadily, don't twist your body too quickly, and try not to make too many sudden movements.

Chapter Six

Sit and Get Fit - Core Training from a Chair

Now it's time to learn the exercises you can do while sitting in a chair. If you're thinking, "Sarah, you don't get it – my mobility isn't what it used to be," I've got your back. This chapter is dedicated to igniting your core from a chair with professionally recognized exercises that are both effective and safe for seniors. Let's get into it!

Seated Marches

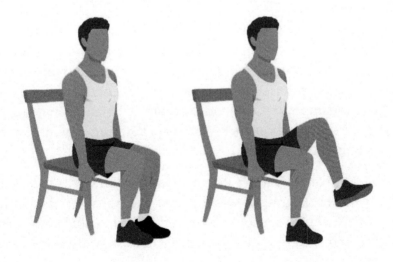

Fig. 6.1

Seated Marches are excellent for engaging your core and improving hip mobility.

Starting Position: Sit up straight towards the edge of your chair with your feet flat on the floor. Keep your shoulders relaxed and your hands resting on your thighs.

Engage Your Core: Pull your navel towards your spine to engage your abdominal muscles.

Lift Your Knee: Lift your right knee towards your chest as high as comfortable, keeping your back straight and avoiding leaning back.

Lower and Repeat: Lower your right foot back to the floor and lift your left knee.

Repeat this alternating motion for 20-30 repetitions (10-15 per leg). This exercise helps to strengthen the lower abdominal muscles and improve overall coordination.

Benefits:

This is a beneficial exercise to incorporate into your routine because it involves the muscles of your lower back and your outer and inner thighs, specifically targeting the core muscles and boosting hip mobility. This exercise is more specific to lower abdomen muscles, but you also improve your coordination and balance. Here are the key benefits you can expect from incorporating Seated Marches into your exercise routine:

1. Core Muscle Activation: Pulling your navel towards your spine keeps your back straight, which works the transverse abdominis and other deep ab muscles. They aid in supporting your spinal column and the groundwork for your core strength and posture improvement.

2. Lower Abdominal Strengthening: When a leg is lifted towards the chest, the lower rectus abdominis muscles, also known as the "lower abs," are pulled and worked on. In most traditional exercise regimens, the lower abs are neglected. However, they're an integral part of your core.

3. Improved Hip Mobility: For efficient performance in Seated Marches, you must smoothly move your hip joints. This exercise is beneficial for anyone who wants to preserve or improve their hip mobility, which is crucial for movement in everyday life, including walking, climbing the stairs, and getting in and out of car seats or chairs.

4. Coordination and Balance: . When you do Seated Marches, you lift one leg at a time and stay straight, so you work on your coordination and balance. Optimizing stability is important for seniors, to help them avoid falls. This exercise will benefit you in this way.

5. Low-Impact Nature: One of the advantages of Seated Marches is that they're very comfortable. Also, they're perfect if you have restricted mobility or an injury. The fact you do it seated means that you don't put pressure on your joints.

As you perform this exercise, be sure to have your back straight and your body posture aligned properly. It is advisable to begin with an acceptable number of repetitions and then raise the intensity bit by bit as the muscles gain strength.

Seated Torso Twists

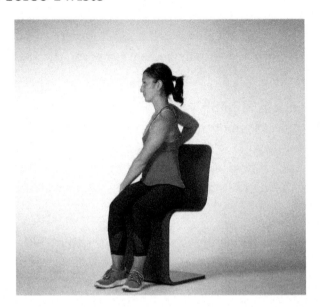

Fig. 6.2a

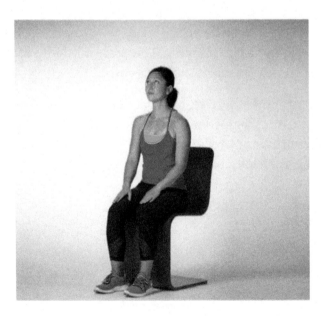

Fig. 6.2b

Seated Torso Twists are great for engaging the obliques and improving spinal mobility.

Starting Position: Sit up straight with your feet flat on the floor, hip-width apart. Extend your arms out in front of you at shoulder height.

Engage Your Core: Pull your navel towards your spine and keep your shoulders relaxed.

Twist to the Right: Slowly twist your torso to the right as far as you can comfortably, keeping your hips stable and your feet planted.

Return to Center: Return to the starting position and then twist to the left.

Perform 15-20 twists on each side. This exercise helps to strengthen the muscles along your sides and improves rotational strength.

Benefits:

Seated Torso Twists are effective for strengthening your oblique muscles and increasing your spine flexibility. This exercise works the oblique muscles of the abdominal region, helping you achieve strength around the belly area and improve your twisting capability. Here are the key benefits you can expect from incorporating Seated Torso Twists into your routine:

1. Oblique Muscle Strengthening: When turning your body side to side, you develop your inner and outer abdominal muscles or the obliques. These muscles are important in rotational movement, postural support, and spine stability.

2. Improved Spinal Mobility: This exercise has an exceptional way of stretching your spine and enhancing flexibility through twisting. The slow turning of the above mass helps provide wider recovery for the thoracic and lumbar spine by improving their

ranges of motion. This can help to relieve back pain and improve spine health.

3. Core Stabilization: Like all exercises that involve twisting, Seated Thoracic Twists target not solely the oblique muscles but also the inner core muscles, including the transverse abdominis and multifidus muscles. These muscles assist in twisting movements by stabilizing your spine and helping to hold it still during this motion.

4. Increased Rotational Strength: Rotation, such as bending down to pick something off the ground, twisting the torso to look behind you, etc., occurs frequently in daily life. Doing Seated Torso Twists can enhance your rotational strength and help prevent injuries when you need to make twisting movements during the day.

5. Low-Impact Nature: Like most seated exercises, Seated Torso Twists are relatively mild, making them quite easy for just about anyone with limited mobility or recovering from an injury. As you do this exercise seated, you don't create joint pressure.

Make sure that you stick to the correct form while doing the exercise, especially if you've got a weak belly. Ensure that your abdominal muscles are taut and that the movements are slow and rhythmic. It is recommended that you begin with a comfortably manageable distance and gradually adjust it over time, as you increase your flexibility and muscle strength.

Seated Leg Extensions

Seated Leg Extensions strengthen the quadriceps and engage the core for stabilization.

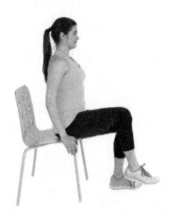

Fig. 6.3a

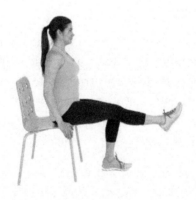

Fig. 6.3b

Starting Position: Sit up straight with your feet flat on the floor, hip-width apart. Place your hands on the sides of the chair for support.

Engage Your Core: Pull your navel towards your spine and maintain a straight back.

Extend Your Right Leg: Slowly extend your right leg out straight in front of you, keeping your foot off the floor.

Hold and Lower: Hold for a few seconds, then lower your leg back down.

Repeat with the left leg and perform 10-15 repetitions on each side. This exercise helps to strengthen the thigh muscles and improve core stability.

Benefits:

Seated leg extensions can be used as a specialized exercise that targets and effectively builds the quadricep and core muscles, which are used to stabilize during the process. This exercise specifically works on the quadricep area in your legs. It is an excellent exercise to strengthen your legs and overall stability.

Here are the key benefits you can expect from incorporating Seated Leg Extensions into your routine:

1. Quadriceps Strengthening: When you try to kick something, push it, or swing your leg, then you work and develop the large muscles that are present on the front side of your thighs, known as the quadricep muscles. In cases of weak knee muscles, some activities affected will be walking, climbing stairs, and standing up from a sitting position.

2. Core Stabilization: The principal function of Seated Leg Extensions is to work the quadriceps, and though the movement may not directly affect the lower back, core muscles are required to stabilize the body during the movement. Holding your belly

button toward your back, you engage your TVA and other stabilizer muscles that support the core tissue, helping you maintain proper spine posture.

3. Improved Leg Mobility: The leg extension movement allows you to adopt a wider array of movements of your leg muscles, including your knee and hip joint flexors, potentially helping to make your legs more flexible.

4. Low-Impact Nature: Seated Leg Extensions are a low-impact exercise. This is good for people with lower mobility, inactive persons, or individuals who are still recuperating from a surgical procedure. You can do this exercise without worrying about making accommodations to avoid joint strain.

5. Versatility: You may want to use different equipment and adding resistance bands or weights to the SE, to work out the corresponding quadriceps muscles.

You can use a low number of repetitions as a starting point and increase them over time, as your muscles get stronger and more flexible.

Seated Side Bends

Seated Side Bends target the obliques and improve flexibility.

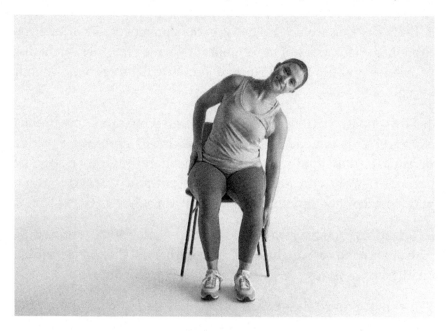

Fig. 6.4

Starting Position: Sit up straight with your feet flat on the floor, hip-width apart. Place your right hand on the side of the chair for support.

Engage Your Core: Pull your navel towards your spine to stabilize your torso.

Reach and Bend: Extend your left arm overhead and bend to the right as far as you can comfortably, feeling the stretch along your left side.

Return to Center: Return to the starting position and switch sides.

Perform 10-15 bends on each side. This exercise enhances lateral flexibility and strengthens the side muscles of the torso.

Benefits:

Sit-ups and side bends are effective for flexing and strengthening the sideway muscles of the abdomen. This exercise targets not only the abdominal muscles and lower back but also the whole spinal unit and body posture.

Here are the key benefits you can expect from incorporating Seated Side Bends into your routine:

1. Oblique Muscle Strengthening: As you sway left and right, you're exercising and building up your muscular body map of internal and external obliques. These muscles are specifically relevant regarding the articulations involving rotation, maintaining core stability, and correct posture.

2. Improved Lateral Flexibility: If these muscles cannot stretch, it will also affect the sides of your body. Hence, this side-bending motion can help stretch these muscles, thereby enhancing the mobility of the torso.

3. Spinal Mobility: This exercise works well on increasing dorsal-spine flexibility, and although the movements are lateral, it offers a great way to initiate the Cordova pushes. This can be very helpful in reducing stiffness and promoting better spinal health.

4. Posture Improvement: Seated Side Bends can also help you achieve a better positioned and postured body, which will help to reduce and prevent back pain.

5. Low-Impact Nature: As the Seated Side Bend is a seated exercise, it's generally easy on the joints and muscles. Also, it's a great choice for people with mobility and/or physical injuries.

Make sure to maintain proper form throughout the exercise, and don't swing your arms too high or force your motions. Remember to control your breathing while performing the exercise, making sure you never end up holding your breath.

Seated Forward Bends

Seated Forward Bends help to stretch the lower back and engage the core.

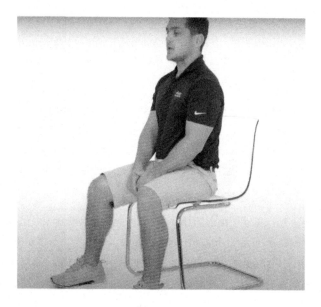

Fig. 6.5a

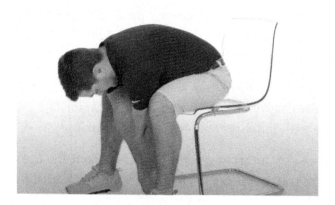

Fig. 6.5b

Starting Position: Sit up straight with your feet flat on the floor, hip-width apart. Extend your arms in front of you at shoulder height.

Engage Your Core: Pull your navel towards your spine and maintain a straight back.

Lean Forward: Slowly lean forward from your hips, reaching down towards your toes while keeping your back straight.

Hold and Return: Hold the forward bend for a few seconds, then return to the starting position.

Repeat this exercise 10-15 times. This movement stretches the lower back and engages the core muscles, promoting flexibility and strength.

Benefits:

Seated Forward Bends are a good exercise to include in programs to increase lower back mobility through stretching and strengthening the abdominal muscles. This exercise is great for encouraging flexibility as well as back, hamstring, and gluteal strength, all of which are part of the posterior chain in the body.

Here are the key benefits you can expect from incorporating Seated Forward Bends into your routine:

1. Lower Back Stretching: That is why, when bending from your hips, you attain a moderate pull on the muscles of your lower back, like the erector spine and the backs of your thighs and hamstrings. This can assist in reducing the tension at times and increase the flexibility in this area.

2. Core Engagement: When leveraging forward, you activate your abdominal muscles to ensure that your spine remains in the correct position and reduce potential stress from the exercise. This exercise strengthens your rectus abdominis—the muscles that form the "V" above your belly button or the "six-pack" muscles—

and your deeper internal support muscles, such as your transverse abdominis.

3. Improved Posture: Seated Forward Bends can improve general posture and even facilitate better spinal structure, decreasing the chance and intensity of back pain and discomfort by developing your abdominal muscles and making the lumbar region more pliant.

4. Hamstring Flexibility: As in any forward bend, Seated Forward Bends are effective in stretching your lower back muscles. They also hit the hamstring muscles, which are the muscles at the back of your thighs. Strengthening these muscles can be useful with preventing leg injuries.

5. Low-Impact Nature: Seated Forward Bends involves gentle and functional movements, which means that they're a good choice for people with minor or severe movement disorders or injuries. While they're a seated exercise, however, you may find them slightly more challenging than others. Be cautious and slow down if you experience any joint pain.

It's important to stay as streamlined as possible while performing all the movements, using your stomach muscles to steady yourself and making your movements deliberate and smooth. Start slow with this exercise, and gradually move further outward as your joint mobility and flexibility improves. Another issue to be careful of is the forward bend. Don't round back; instead, bend from your lower abdomen area.

Seated Russian Twists

Seated Russian Twists are a great way to engage the obliques and improve rotational strength.

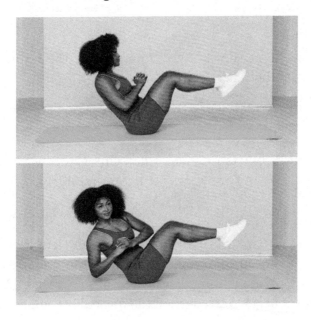

Fig. 6.6a

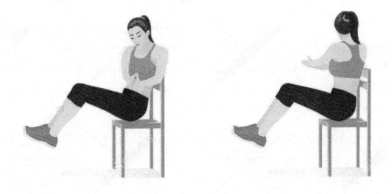

Fig. 6.6b

Starting Position: Sit up straight with your feet flat on the floor, hip-width apart. Extend your arms in front of you, clasping your hands together.

Engage Your Core: Pull your navel towards your spine and keep your shoulders relaxed.

Twist to the Right: Slowly twist your torso to the right, bringing your hands to the side of your body.

Return to Center: Return to the starting position and then twist to the left.

Perform 10-15 twists on each side. This exercise targets your oblique muscles and enhances your core stability.

Benefits:

Seated Russian Twists are one of the most efficient exercises that work effectively to tone and strengthen the oblique and core muscles. This exercise directly involves muscles at the sides of your torso. Also, it helps to strengthen the muscular endurance in your limbs.

Here are the key benefits you can expect from incorporating Seated Russian Twists into your routine:

1. Oblique Muscle Strengthening: Every time you twist your upper body one way and the other, you work on both your internal and external oblique muscles. They're involved in rotation, stabilization, and positional strength, including the attachments between the spine and the lower limbs.

2. Improved Rotational Strength: Some of the routine functional movements that involve using your rotational strength include stretching or flexing to get an object or shifting in a chair to look at what is behind you. Introducing Seated Russian Twists into your

regular fitness practices will let you build up the ability to carry out these functions more safely and easily.

3. Core Stabilization: Seated Russian twists primarily target your obliques. Also, they help work your secondary stabilizer muscles, the transverse abdominis and multifidus muscles. Some of these muscles support the spine, while others act as a base that supports the backbone during the twisting.

4. Balance and Coordination: Rotary crunch involves twisters that have to be done in a balanced manner. They require strict body stability to enable the twirling of the torso. This can enhance the subject's ability to understand body position and locate it in space, as well as the ability to exert control over the body.

5. Low-Impact Nature: Seated Russian Twists are a low-impact exercise, and they come in handy especially if the person has a limited range of motion or has an injury. The exercise can be done while seated, posing no strain on the joints or muscles.

Keep your posture straight and maintain control of your movements as you do Seated Russian Twists. It is wise to begin the session with a comfortable range of motion and gradually get to the next level of difficulty as your flexibility and the strength improve. Make sure that you don't accidentally hold your breath while doing this exercise.

Seated Crunches:

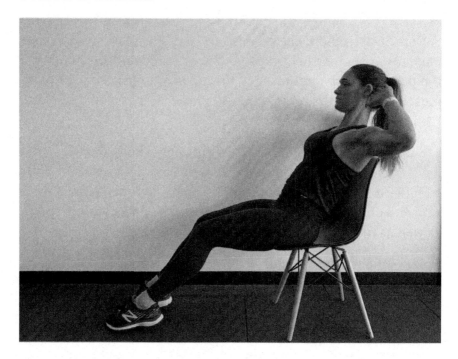

Fig. 6.7

Seated Crunches are an excellent exercise for strengthening your core without the need to lie on the floor. This exercise targets your abdominal muscles, helping to improve your overall core strength and stability.

Starting Position: Sit on the edge of a chair with your hands placed behind your head. Lightly balance your toes on the ground to maintain stability.

Engage Your Core: Pull your navel towards your spine to engage your lower core muscles.

Lean Back: Slowly lean your torso back towards the chair, maintaining a straight spine throughout the movement.

Crunch Forward: Once you've leaned back comfortably, crunch back up by bringing your torso forward. Ensure your movements are controlled and deliberate.

Repeat: Perform 15-20 repetitions of this exercise, focusing on engaging your core and maintaining proper form.

Benefits:

People can strengthen their abdominal muscles in Seated Crunches without risking falling over. It is a highly effective exercise. It should help to enhance your general muscular strength, particularly when it comes to the core muscles.

Here are the key benefits you can expect from incorporating Seated Crunches into your routine:

1. Rectus Abdominis Strengthening: As you advance, it is the rectus abdominis muscles or the 'six-pack' muscles that you activate and tone. These muscles offer lumbar stability, which is crucial in helping you maintain correct posture and making you less likely to develop backache.

2. Oblique Muscle Activation: While the rectus abdominis is the primary muscle worked on through Seated Crunches, the movements also involve the oblique muscles (the muscles located on the side of the abdomen). These muscles are innervated to aid in the rotational movement of the spine and play a vital role as stabilizers.

3. Improved Breathing Mechanics: Seated Crunches, when done in a controlled and safe manner, can also help you use the diaphragm properly and beneficially influence many aspects of breathing mechanics. This will ultimately increase your internal and external coordination and help you function in coordination with your routine activities.

4. Low-Impact Nature: Seated Crunches can also be considered the most convenient movement since they're low-impact and suitable for people with mobility issues or health problems. This exercise is quite comfortable when done while seated, so minimal pressure is put on the joints.

5. Versatility: As with most exercises involving lying on your back, Seated Crunches can be made even more difficult by incorporating resistance bands or weights to effectively punch away at your abdominal muscles from all angles. Alternatively, to make the exercise more complicated, you could change the angle of the movement or speed, helping to strengthen the core muscles even more.

As a reminder, the next time you do this exercise, maintain good posture to get the most out of the move while protecting your neck and lower back from injury. It is critical to safeguard the abs, limit the motion, and refrain from tugging on the neck with your hands. The number of repetitions should be chosen for comfort and you can increase them later, after you build strength.

Chapter Seven

The Standing Core Workout

I'm so happy you're still here! I really appreciate your effort and commitment to strengthening your core. Now it's time for the next evolution, my friend. As a change, we'll include some standing core exercises in our training schedule! Standing core workouts are excellent for building strength, improving balance, and engaging your muscles in a functional way. Let's dive in!

Standing Side Bends

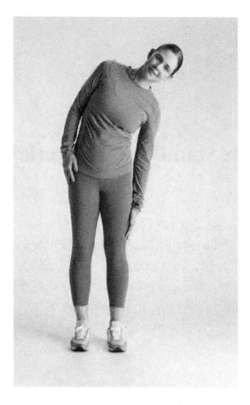

Fig. 7.1

Side bends help strengthen your oblique muscles, which are crucial for core stability. This exercise also improves flexibility in your sides.

Instructions:

1. Starting Position: Stand with your feet shoulder-width apart, and place your hands on your hips.

2. Action: Slowly bend to the right side, reaching your right hand down your leg. Return to the center and then bend to the left.

3. Reps: Perform 10 bends on each side.

Tips:

- Keep your movements slow and controlled to maximize the stretch and engagement.

- Ensure your upper body remains straight and does not lean forward or backward.

- Breathe steadily and deeply throughout the exercise.

Benefits:

The Standing Side Bend is an outstanding oblique exercise, as it helps the muscles on the side of the abdominal wall stabilize the core and perform rotation movements. The sides of your torso will become more flexible, helping to enhance mobility.

Here are the key benefits you can expect from incorporating Standing Side Bends into your routine:

1. Oblique Muscle Strengthening: When swaying from the right to the left side, you tone and develop your internal and external oblique muscles. These muscles are important in rotational activities, torsional strength, and body postural control.

2. Improved Lateral Flexibility: This exercise's side-bending motion assists in stretching tissues on either side of the torso, which would help increase mobility and flexibility around the torso area.

3. Spinal Mobility: I found out that Standing Side Bends are effective in stretching different muscles in the body, especially on the lateral plane of the spine. This can be useful in reducing feelings of stiffness, and this kind of adjustment will also boost the spine's health.

4. Posture Improvement: Besides preventing and alleviating pain in the oblique muscles and lower back, the improvement in spinal flexibility resulting from Standing Side Bends also helps to prevent excessive slouching and possible resultant back ache or pain.

5. Low-Impact Nature: Standing Side Bends are an effective exercise for weight loss while still being low-impact. They can be appropriate for many people with illnesses and injuries.

It is imperative to ensure that you maintain proper form and posture throughout the exercise, with your tummy muscles tightened and smooth. Make sure that your movements are controlled. Perform the repetitions and sets as long as you comfortably can, starting with a good amount of flexibility and gradually progressing through the set as toning increases. It should also be noted that you should adhere to a constant breathing technique and avoid taking deep breaths.

Hip Circle Exercise

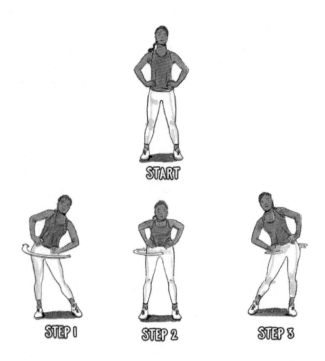

Fig. 7.2

The Hip Circle exercise is excellent for warming up your hips, improving flexibility, and enhancing the range of motion in your hip joints. This exercise targets the muscles around the hips, including the glutes, hip flexors, and abductors.

Instructions:

Starting Position:

- Stand with your feet shoulder-width apart and place your hands on your hips.

- Engage your core by pulling your belly button towards your spine.

Action:

- Slowly move your hips in a circular motion, starting from the right side.

- Complete a full circle by moving your hips forward, to the left, backward, and then back to the starting position.

- After completing a set of circles in one direction, reverse the direction and perform the same number of circles.

Reps: Perform 10 hip circles in each direction.

Tips:

- Keep your movements slow and controlled to maximize the stretch and engagement of your hip muscles.

- Ensure your upper body remains still and does not lean forward or backward.

- Breathe steadily and deeply throughout the exercise.

Benefits:

The Hip Circle Exercise is another wonderful tool that will help you with the hip's warming up, increasing flexibility, and increasing hip joint mobility. This exercise basically involves the contraction of the hip's circular muscles, such as the gluteus, hip flexor, and hip abductor muscles.

Here are the key benefits you can expect from incorporating Hip Circle Exercise into your routine:

1. Increased Hip Flexibility: Circular hip motion engages the hip muscles directly and indirectly, meaning you increase the flexibility of muscles around those joints, such as the gluteus, hip flexors, and abductors.

2. Improved Range of Motion: The circular motion in this exercise also facilitates stretching of the hip joints, thereby improving global flexibility and minimizing the likelihood of getting hurt while exercising or at work.

3. Muscle Activation: However, before concentrating the heat on the muscles around the hips, the Hip Circle Exercise also targets specific muscles in that area to prepare for other vigorous exercise routines.

4. Warm-up Preparation: The Hip Circle exercise is a warm-up activity for your regular workout. It prepares the muscles and joints in your hips for activity, enhancing your chances of preventing injury during your exercise.

5. Low-Impact Nature: Just like any Standing Exercise, the Hip Circle exercise does not demand much stress on the joints. That means it can be done by people with different problems or recovering from injuries.

Remember to maintain correct posture throughout the exercise, with the tummy muscles pulled in and smooth movements made. Use the given starting flexibility and gradually progress towards a better range as you continue with the exercises. Make sure that your breathing is consistent and regular.

Standing Torso Twist

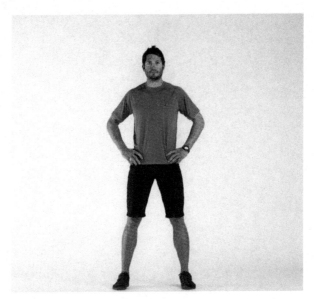

Fig. 7.3a

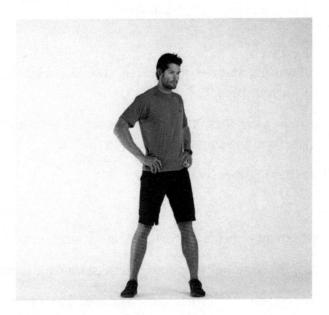

Fig. 7.3b

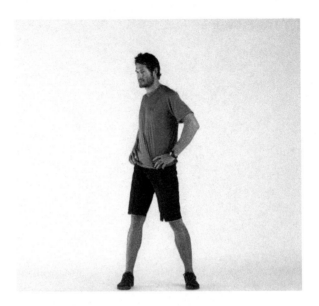

Fig. 7.3c

This exercise is great for your oblique muscles and overall core strength. It also improves spinal mobility.

Instructions:

1. Starting Position: Stand with your feet shoulder-width apart and your hands on your hips.

2. Action: Twist your torso to the right, keeping your hips facing forward. Return to the center and twist to the left.

3. Reps: Do this 10 times on each side.

Tips:

- Make sure your movements are controlled and your core remains tight.

- Keep your hips stationary to focus the twist on your torso.

- Breathe out as you twist to each side and breathe in as you return to the center.

Benefits:

Doing this exercise will help your strength and flexibility for lateral bends. Also, it's highly effective in creating stability throughout your torso and spine. This exercise targets the velocity of the muscles of your abdomen, not only your outer abdominal muscles but your inner abdominal muscles as well. Additionally, it helps increase the flexibility of your rotational muscles.

Here are the key benefits you can expect from incorporating Standing Torso Twists into your routine:

1. Oblique Muscle Strengthening: Twisting from your waist sideways lets you work on your internal and external oblique muscles. It fixates itself to the spine and plays significant roles in rotational movements, core support, and body alignment.

2. Improved Spinal Mobility: The bending in this particular exercise helps to increase the flexibility and mobility of the spine in the rotational plane. It may help to reduce built-up stiffness and promote better health of the spinal cord.

3. Core Stabilization: Though categorized as an oblique workout, Standing Torso Twists are a bonus for your deep core muscles, including the transverse abdominis and multifidus muscles. These muscles help maintain the stability of your spinal column during torsion.

4. Increased Rotational Strength: Since most of us perform rotational movements in our daily activities, like reaching out for an object or turning around to look behind, spinal rotation is an important function. As you add Standing Torso Twists to your workout regimen, you'll gain higher and greater tropical strength, hence having less inclination to get injured in these movements.

5. Low-Impact Nature: Standing Torso Twists don't put excessive stress on the joints, which is why they're suitable for people with

low fitness levels, as well as for injured athletes who are taking time off from heavy training.

Make sure that you maintain proper posture throughout this exercise. This includes engaging the stomach muscle and making smooth and orderly movements. This is a low-impact stretching exercise, but you must still ensure you start with a comfortable position. Perform the exercise to a level that is appropriate for your comfort and flexibility. Keep your breathing regular, and make sure you never inadvertently hold your breath.

Knee Lifts

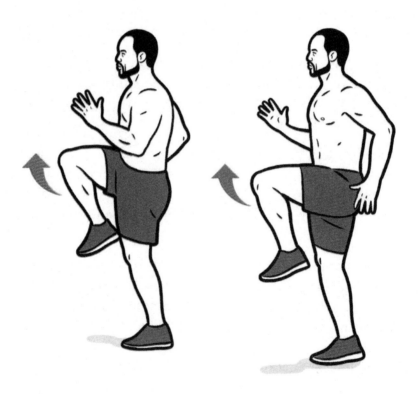

Fig. 7.4

Knee lifts target the lower abs and improve balance. They're simple yet effective for engaging your core muscles.

Instructions:

1. Starting Position: Stand tall with your feet hip-width apart.

2. Action: Lift your right knee towards your chest and lower it back down. Repeat with your left knee.

3. Reps: Do this 10 times on each side.

Tips:

- Keep your back straight and engage your core throughout the movement.

- Move slowly and with control to maximize the engagement of your core muscles.

- To increase the challenge, lift your knees higher or hold each knee lift for a few seconds.

Benefits:

The Knee Lift is a basic and safe exercise that strengthens and tones the Six-Pack Abs muscle zone. It helps to improve your balance, as well. This variant strengthens my abdominal muscles and tests my spatial awareness and balance. Here are the key benefits you can expect from incorporating Knee Lifts into your routine:

1. Lower Abdominal Strengthening: During the movement, when you're holding your knees near your chest, your lower rectus abdominis muscles, also known as the 'lower abs,' are being worked out. This component of abdominal strength plays a crucial role in several ab exercises.

2. Improved Balance and Coordination: Swinging one leg while standing is an effective way of stretching the lower limbs. Since

you stand upright while doing it, you feel able to test your balance and coordination. This exercise can enhance overall stability and it may be useful in maintaining the balance of older people, potentially improving their functional mobility and reducing the likelihood of falls.

3. Core Engagement: Knee Lifts primarily work on your lower ab muscles, but they're not selective of your core muscles: they hit the transverse abdominis and multifidus. These muscles synchronize to stabilize your spine during the exercise.

4. Low-Impact Nature: Knee Lifts are easy on the joints, so most people can do them safely at varying levels of intensity.

5. Versatility: When you feel ready, you can adjust Knee Lifts to be more challenging by raising the legs to a higher level, holding the Lifts for a longer time, and/or incorporating bands and weights.

It's crucial to maintain proper posture throughout the exercise and ensure you contract your abdominal muscles while minimizing jerky movements. Begin with a set that you feel comfortable with, and then, as your muscle strength and stamina increase, you can try a higher repetition set. Keep your breathing regular.

Standing Elbow to Knee

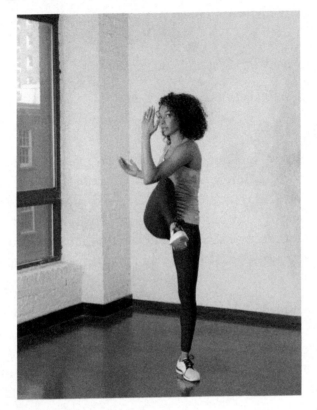

Fig. 7.5

This exercise combines a bit of cardio with core strengthening. It targets the oblique muscles and improves balance and coordination.

Instructions:

1. Starting Position: Stand with your feet shoulder-width apart and your hands behind your head.

2. Action: Lift your right knee and try to touch it with your left elbow. Lower your knee and repeat with the opposite side.

3. Reps: Perform 10 touches on each side.

Tips:

- Move slowly and with control to maximize the engagement of your core muscles.

- Keep your back straight and your core tight.

- Breathe steadily throughout the exercise.

Benefits:

Standing Elbow to Knee is another great exercise that involves balance, core stability, and full-body coordination alongside the cardiovascular component. This exercise focuses on the development of your oblique muscular region and, at the same time, strengthening balance and coordination. Here are the key benefits you can expect from incorporating Standing Elbow to Knee:

1. Oblique Muscle Strengthening: When you attempt to grab your knee with the opposite elbow while lifting the knee, you're flexing and thus exercising your internal and external oblique muscles. These muscles are important in rotational movements of the upper body, postural support and stability, and shoulder girdle movements.

2. Improved Balance and Coordination: Swing your leg up and down and, at the same time, extend your hand with your elbow, creating a tough regimen for your balance and coordination. These are exercises that may also be of value in training your body awareness and, therefore, help prevent falls and enhance your movements on the floor.

3. Cardio Component: Although it is not an ostensive cardiovascular exercise, due to the active engagement of several body parts during Standing Elbow to Knee, the heart rate could be slightly raised, and hence, it does have a low-impact cardio aspect in the progression of the activity.

4. Core Stabilization: Standing Elbow to Knee holds significant cues and affects the muscle layer beneath the external ones, including the transverse abdominis and the multifidus. These muscles act in coordination with the twisting motion, to support and stabilize.

5. Low-Impact Nature: Standing Elbow to Knee is a relatively easy exercise since most body parts don't come into contact with the ground. Thus, the impact is low and preferred by people with low fitness or those with injury cases.

Maintaining good posture and form during this exercise is important, keeping the stomach tight and moving slowly and deliberately. It is advisable to begin with a manageable number of repetitions and eventually add to them as the muscles get stronger and the duration of repetition increases. Make sure you keep your breathing regular as you exercise, making sure that you never hold your breath.

Side Leg Lifts

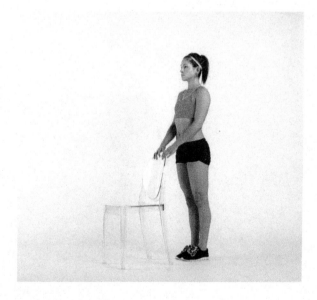

Fig. 7.6a

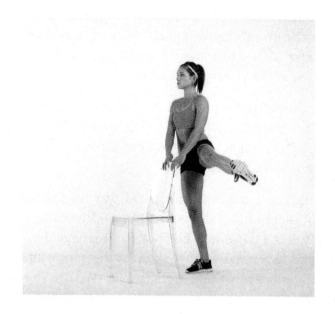

Fig. 7.6b

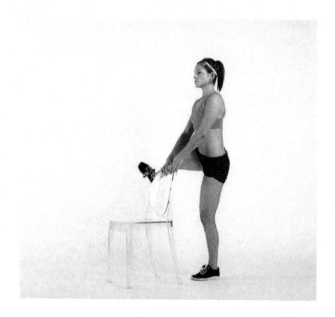

Fig. 7.6c

Side Leg Lifts help strengthen the muscles on the sides of your core, known as the obliques. They also improve hip flexibility and stability.

Instructions:

1. Starting Position: Stand with your feet shoulder-width apart and your hands on your hips.

2. Action: Lift your right leg out to the side and lower it back down. Repeat with your left leg.

3. Reps: Do this 10 times on each side.

Tips:

- Keep your upper body straight and avoid leaning to the side.

- Move slowly and with control to maximize the engagement of your core muscles.

- To increase the challenge, hold each leg lift for a few seconds.

Benefits:

Side Leg Lifts benefit your tummy, particularly the muscles that lie to the side of your belly, referred to as the obliques. They also improve hip flexibility and stability. Since this exercise focuses on twisting moves, it is ideal for strengthening the obliques, hip flexors, and abductors, boosting the overall core strength and flexibility.

Here are the key benefits you can expect from incorporating Side Leg Lifts into your routine:

1. Oblique Muscle Strengthening: When you move your leg out to the side, your internal and external oblique muscles are used as you lift the leg. These muscles are involved in most movements involving rotation and support to the overpowering muscles.

2. Hip Flexor and Abductor Strengthening: If performed correctly, Side Leg Lifts directly hit the obliques and tone your hip flexors and abductors. Your hip flexors and abductors are crucial for tasks such as climbing stairs and sustaining proper posture. They're key to stabilization and injury prevention.

3. Improved Hip Flexibility: The lateral leg movement in this exercise also works the hip joints, and therefore, it is important that the hips can flex and move laterally to the extent needed for the exercise. Side Leg Lifts help strengthen our hip muscles, making them more flexible. Start slowly with this exercise, building up to doing more as you progress from day to day. Don't push yourself too hard. 4. Core Stabilization: Side leg lifts give you an impressive workout. They target your obliques, hip muscles, and deep core muscles, including the transverse abdominis and multifidus muscles. These muscles act in synergy and help support the spine whenever you perform this kind of exercise.

5. Low-Impact Nature: Side Leg Lifts help strengthen the muscles of the hip, thigh, and buttocks as well as the lower abdominal area, without putting too much pressure on the knees or back. This is why they're a good pick for many beginning exercisers and those with limited mobility or injuries.

Make sure you maintain the correct form during this exercise. You should engage your abdominal muscles and move slowly and steadily. Begin with the easiest pose on the floor and introduce little variations as the muscles become more flexible. Keep up a steady breathing pattern.

Standing Plank

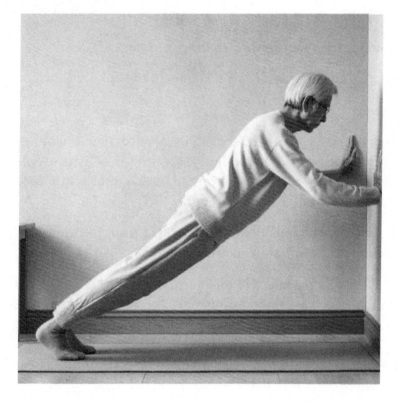

Fig. 7.7

The Standing Plank mimics the traditional plank but in a standing position. It's great for engaging your entire core while also improving balance.

Instructions:

1. Starting Position: Stand facing a wall, and place your hands on the wall at shoulder height.

2. Action: Walk your feet back until your body forms a straight line from head to heels.

3. Hold: Hold this position for 30 seconds.

Tips:

- Engage your core and keep your body in a straight line.

- Avoid sagging your hips or arching your back.

- Breathe steadily and deeply throughout the hold.

Benefits:

Standing Plank is an intermediate-level exercise where your posture resembles a plank, but you're standing. This exercise is particularly useful when you want to work out the entire core and develop better balance and strength.

Here are the key benefits you can expect from incorporating the Standing Plank into your routine:

1. Full Core Engagement: While normal planking exercises mainly focus on the rectus abdominis muscles, also referred to as the front abs, the Standing Plank equally involves the exterior abs and the posterior abs, as well as the lower back muscles known as the erector spinae muscles. This full-body activation can directly benefit the core muscular structure and enhance core stability.

2. Improved Balance and Proprioception: By holding a plank pose while standing, you exercise your balance as well as proprioception (the knowledge of the location and movement of individual body parts). This exercise can be useful in enhancing steadiness, balance, and proprioception, which are critical for optimal mobility without falls.

3. Spinal Alignment: The Standing Plank involves straight alignment from the head to the heels, and it increases your awareness of body position and spinal posture. It can be highly effective for individuals who spend much of their time in a chair (for example, people who drive for a living or spend most of their day at a desk).

4. Versatility: You can easily ramp up or tone down the Standing Plank by modifying your stance (that is, narrow stance or wide stance) and adding some dynamics that include the arms or legs. Alternatively, you could even add intensity with accessories, such as resistance bands or some free weights.

5. Low-Impact Nature: Like most standing exercises, the Standing Plank is relatively safer than high-impact exercises. Thus, it can be performed by a broad category of people, including those in the early stages of training and even individuals with certain kinds of injuries.

Remember to maintain proper form and posture while performing this exercise, specifically by keeping your stomach muscles tight and your back straight. Begin with an intermediate hold time and then work your way up as your body gets stronger and more accustomed to the exercise. Make sure to keep your breathing regular when you're doing the Standing Plank.

Chapter Eight

Cool Down

Give yourself a moment to sit back and enjoy your post-exercise high. Those muscles are buzzing, that heart is beating, you're all sweaty and a little shiny. It's all the encouragement we need!

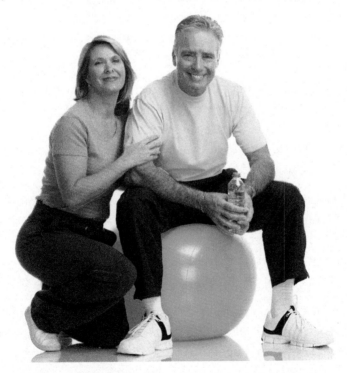

Fig. 8.1

Hydration Celebration:

After a good exercise session, don't forget to rehydrate. You need to replace the water you sweated out! Despite this being a relatively low-intensity workout, rehydration is a vital component of the recovery process. So, let's celebrate your efforts with plenty of delicious, cold water.

Give yourself time to savor the water as you give your body the hydration it needs. When you take the first gentle draught, let the liquid run freely on the tongue. Can you feel your body buzzing with energy at that first refreshing sip? It's like a parched plant that can finally reap the benefits of the first rain.

Take it down with purpose. Try to savor the taste and visualize the drink replenishing your overworked muscles. Imagine that stream of hydration going throughout your body and feeding those cells, rejuvenating them and cleaning out waste and lactic acid. It's like getting a new, fresh start!

I'd like you to enjoy these purposeful sips and drink slowly, taking in each refreshing mouthful of this ultra-hydrating drink. As you refill your water bottle, be mindful. Take your time and be as conscious as possible of the process. Make sure you replenish yourself with at least 16 ounces before you call it a day.

But if you get tired of drinking just plain water, go ahead and add some excitement! If you're using a glass, you could garnish it with some mint leaves, cucumber, or orange slices. Don't forget the ice! You could even add a pinch of electrolyte powder or True Lemon seasoning to enhance the energy-boosting properties.

Personally, I prefer to stir in a few ounces of 100% fruit juice for its sweetness. It's delicious and looks like a non-alcoholic cocktail! The only garnish that accompanies my glass of grapefruit juice is lime. It's amazing after a good workout session.

It's important to drink the recommended daily water intake, but you don't have to stick to plain water. Get creative with how you'll enjoy the process! Plus, accompany your water with other things that you enjoy, like listening to your favorite song, enjoying a few chapters of the novel you've been enjoying, or catching up on a conversation with a friend. Hydration celebration, baby!

Talking about celebrations, there's one more factor to include to enhance the recovery process and wake up the fat burner within. It's a step count challenge!

Step Count Challenge:

You've put so much effort into working your core muscles, you don't want to spend the rest of the day on the couch. Let's keep on feeding that metabolism furnace!

It's time to get your steps in, but no need to worry. You can do it in a fun way! Remember, staying active is crucial for keeping your joints flexible, so they don't seize up or restrict you. Even if you just take a ten-minute stroll around the neighborhood, every motion matters, no matter how insignificant it may seem!

The best part? You've already in exercise mode. So don't break the pace. If you want, you can just walk around your house or backyard. You'll help maintain your joint lubrication, and the steps will add up before you know it. Win-win!

Plus, walking around can be your cool down. Remember, you've just done a workout. Don't suddenly bring everything to a standstill. Go for a leisurely walk through the park or a nature trail and breathe in the fresh air. It's also possible to supplement your walk with standing stretches every few minutes to improve your flexibility.

Not only will you get a great step count in without even knowing it, but being outdoors and breathing in the fresh air will help your body recover. This is my favorite post-workout remedy!

But what if you don't want to go outside? Well, you can just walk around your living room or hallway, maybe sometimes stopping to do stretch exercises. A few minor tasks, such as walking from one room to another with a laundry basket, can also help maintain a steady step count. Indeed, any kind of movement is the name of the game here.

The best part? The extra steps you log today don't have to be an all-or-nothing marathon. A series of micro-step sessions is as effective in burning calories and lubricating the joints as a single session of more prolonged and intense walking. So, get in the habit of incorporating more movement into your day whenever possible.

Challenge yourself (ever so slightly) – try to do 2,000 more steps than you usually do in a day. Maybe even 10,000 if you feel particularly adventurous today. You can use a wearable pedometer or a smartphone app to track your progress. Every step is a reason to cheer!

The focus is staying mobile and improving blood circulation. No need to go for high-intensity zones here. Think soft-serve ice cream with warm pie topping rather than anything more exotic.

By the time you're done hydrating and have achieved your steps for the day, I can almost bet my last dollar that you'll feel more rejuvenated than you did when the day started. This is where the magic happens, so to speak—all these cool-down movements can help you enhance the impact of your core workout!

Chapter Nine

Pro Tips for Max Core Benefits

If you've reached this stage in our core strengthening journey, I know you're an outstanding, hardworking star. That takes a lot of tenacity and determination, so congratulations!

But by now, you might be looking forward to having new ideas and approaches that will make this core training exciting again. Even the most effective exercises can become monotonous when we feel like we're just going through the motions and not feeling engaged.

Don't worry, my hardworking friend! You're in luck because here I'll give you a tasty menu of invigorating ideas that will spice up your core work in rather unexpected ways. We're discussing some of the cool ways to step up your engagement, some of the unique workout features, and a little bit of silly additions as well. And this brings us to the final point— at the end of the day, fitness should absolutely be fun.

Here are the final steps of learning that I've gathered in understanding the keys to successful exercise motivation over the years. You've done the work – now, it's time to add more character and enjoyment to each activity!

Well, you know what they say—all that core work isn't going to do itself. It takes a lot of energy, so grab a snack, perhaps take a notepad and pen, and let's get your core training on the right track. The best is yet to come.

1) Letting Go

Remember when you were a kid, and you played with your friends? You were just having fun! There weren't any rigid rules. Perhaps it was playing pretend when you were racing your toy car around the backyard, or when you were thought you were a superhero playing with friends in the neighborhood. Whatever it was, I'm sure that you were fully absorbed in that happy state of being with no care in the world about calorie-burning or muscle-toning.

Oh well, I've good news for you—that childlike spirit of fun is still there inside you, patiently waiting for the opportunity to come out and play! So, if you want to inject new life and sustainability into your training, call on your inner child to inspire you during your core routines.

It may be as basic as wearing outrageous costume props or pretending to be a character. Maybe you'll put on an eye patch and a peg leg and pretend to be a pirate during the standing core exercise and shout 'arrs' with each repetition! Or maybe you'd prefer wearing a wild wig and glittery scarf and pretend to be your favorite disco-dancing diva while doing hip circles.

You could even have a storytelling session where you tell the story of the exercises. A particular client of mine used to pretend she was a tiny, skinny scientist dealing with the inside world of her body every time she had to do core work. "And here we're in the oblique canyon. . . better engage those external abdominal obliques for stability as we descend into the depths!" A little ridiculous? Sure. But you won't get bored!

These are simple and more complex ideas to get more playful – the options are virtually limitless. All you need is to get back in touch with the curiosity and creativity you had as a child. These goofy tricks will help you stay energetic and interested and get you straight into that wonderful state of presence you're looking for. Developing your inner child will be so entertaining, you might even forget that you're exercising!

2) Gamify Your Experience

Keeping with that silly tone, another great strategy to intensify your core training excitement is to make it fun and turn it into a game. Most people are intrinsically competitive, and we're driven by the need to pursue interesting things in life. Why not take advantage of that innate need for enjoyable challenges?

This is one of the most engaging gamification strategies that I recommend to anyone looking to add a competitive edge to a project: the element of surprise. For instance, you could write down 10-15 of the core movements that you prefer on separate pieces of paper, mix them in a hat, and then perform the movements in the order that you randomly pull them out. You can call this your "core routine lottery." This way, you'll be able to have more fun and bring a new focus to your core workouts.

You can crank it up by assigning different points for the different moves or exercise 'taxes' to pay when a specific one is drawn. For example, bicycles might be worth 5 points, while hollow body holds are worth 20 points. Assign a total point target to strive to achieve each time you train, and get ready to witness your core engage like never before as you try to hit the mark!

If you live with family or friends, you could turn it into a full-on core competition by partnering up. Split the players into two groups and take turns picking cards for the exercise draws, with each team gaining points for the cards chosen while attempting to choose difficult moves for the other team whenever possible.

Some fitness apps and video games make it easy to keep track of your progress. Some are equipped with encouraging incentives like gaining points, achieving levels, getting bonuses, or reaching new worlds as you frequently record exercises. You could target to pulverize weekly step targets or count enough activity minutes for an exciting virtual hiking trail.

Regardless of how you decide to apply game-ification to your core training, the idea is to add a wildcard element of fun and incentive so that you're chasing those happy juice feels with the fierce determination of a hamster on a wheel. It's always great to enjoy a keen sense of accomplishment, even triumph!

3) Add Joy With Music And Lighting

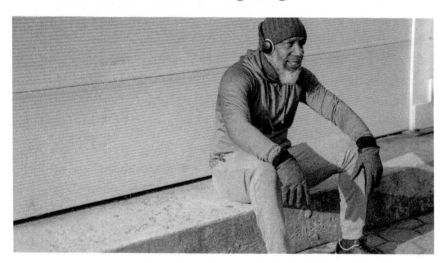

Fig. 9.1

If you've stayed with me on this core strengthening exercise journey, you know by now that your mindset is very powerful in the kind of results you get. That is true with any kind of exercise. All good things come to those ready to work with the right attitude, energy, enthusiasm, and an open mind.

One of the best pieces of advice I can give when it comes to making long-term, positive changes in your exercise routine is to bring positivity, including music and atmosphere, wherever possible. Our surroundings have more influence than you probably imagine in influencing our feelings, and even our hormonal balance. Create an atmosphere to foster a feeling of optimism and happiness.

Think about putting together a mood-enhancing music playlist customized to your taste. It can make all the difference in the world. Make sure to include all the best feel-good songs that you want to belt out at the top of your lungs. The ones with powerful voices, inspirational messages, or simple contagious grooves that makes your head nod in approval.

Then, make it an ultra-high priority to press play and crank those tunes during every core session! Don't just use this as background music. Instead, make sure to truly feel the rhythm and beat in your body while breathing and dancing. Sing if you want, make your mini-dance moves between sets, or even make up lyrics about how much muscle you're building!

The physical changes that come with synchronizing the workout to a motivating playlist are not to be taken lightly. At the most fundamental level, the increased tempo of the song and the uplifting words that are sung convey invigorating messages that trigger pleasure points in the brain. Consequently, you'll naturally gain better coordination, desire, and focus on the present—a total vibe!

However, as great as this approach may be, there are several other methods you can try to enhance the happy atmosphere.. You may enjoy using stimulating scents such as grapefruit or eucalyptus during your workout to give you a calming yet exciting boost. Maybe you'd like to invest in an essential oil diffuser. Or you can light a scented candle within the workout area to create a new layer of atmosphere. Other options include using Himalayan salt lamps, string lights, or even just turning off the overhead lights and fixtures. Just make sure you can see properly.

If you want to transport yourself to another world, why not get kitschy and set up a thematic backdrop or scenery cues for your routines? For instance, you could put up some beach wallpaper prints and spray a weak salt air fragrance that would make you feel like you're on the beach as you perform your core work. Random? Yes. Fun and memorable? Absolutely!

In other words, we always train better when we have a positive mindset. That's why you should imagine how you can infuse more positivity into the actions you perform each day, thinking of all five senses. Spoiler alert: It will be great – those endorphins will be off the charts!

4) Embrace the Weird

Sticking with that fun and funky theme, my final piece of premium core training advice is this: let yourself go all out and never feel guilty about being awkward or strange! Because at a certain stage, avoiding looking and feeling awkward or silly during exercise is impossible if you want to give your best effort.

Imagine that – we're often bending our spines in rather awkward and inconvenient ways during core exercises, are we not? Maybe we almost feel like we're scooting around like pretzels, scrunching up like little balls, and perching delicately on our fleshy sit bones! Sometimes, I think it would be strange if we did not consider ourselves somewhat ridiculous at least once in a while!

Instead of getting embarrassed or uncomfortable about those moments that are naturally silly, go ahead and embrace them. Laugh at yourself in the mirror as you struggle to pull off an awkward dance move. Some exercises may have seemed quite difficult a few weeks ago, so do a little shimmy shake when you get a few reps. Well done, you! It's time for some applause as you get through those plank series!

Here's the real deal: you need to embrace your flaws and be ready to be as cringe-worthy as possible whenever necessary. First, this will do away with any lingering shyness or self-consciousness, and worry about looking foolish. It's difficult to overestimate how liberating it can be to set aside your worries and let loose. You'll find that you challenge yourself in the best possible ways when you set aside your fears of criticism.

You'll find it much easier to let yourself off the hook to experiment with new movements with wonder rather than fear. This creates a fun, whimsical, and wonderfully peculiar feeling! On the surface, you're taking the whole experience much less seriously, but you are becoming much more invested on a more meaningful level.

I remember once seeing someone make funny little hissy cat imitations at the end of her core finishers when she felt pain. Sometimes, she just made a funny face and hummed silly "tsssssss" sounds as the reps became more painful. And you know what? It made the discomfort feel like a new fun game, and the blowing also boosted her breath support!

So, it's time to get truly creative. I urge you to look for your own unique ways of embracing the weirdness involved in core training. You can rate your quivering muscles on a silliness scale of 1 to 10. Go ahead and howl like a wolf, yelp like a dog, or even purr like a cat if that puts you in the right state of mind! This is something that I've often heard people say, but I never really understood how important it was.

And you might even encourage others to take the same approach, for their own good. Imagine a crew of dedicated core weirdos to train, share laughter, and become even stronger with!

Chapter Ten

Simple Diet Wins

Nourishing Your Core

As we've looked at core strengthening and flexible movements, we've encountered several ways to create a stronger and younger-looking body. However, as any builder will attest, a strong home requires a good foundation and regular feeding to support and maintain the structure. From this chapter onwards, we shift from physical activities to what we put in our bodies to provide energy for such exercises – food. The food we eat is a key determinant of the foundational strength we're building. Let's make healthy and delicious foods part of your daily routine. Are you ready to explore the world of food and nutrition? Let's go!

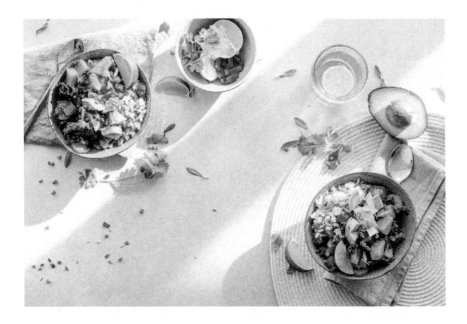

Fig. 10.1

1. Feeding Your Core: Basics of a Core-Friendly Diet

Remember that physical exercise isn't the only factor that contributes to a strong core. The food you eat also has a major impact. You should select foods that are not only delicious but also promote muscle recovery and energy endurance. Examples include chicken, turkey, tofu, and legumes. These proteins help with muscle building, which is as important as the exercises we did in Chapter 4. Quinoa, brown rice, and other whole grains give us the slow-burning energy to keep us going, while a wide selection of vegetables and fruits gives us the vitamins and antioxidants we need.

Tip: Embrace variety! Just as we should avoid monotony with our workouts, it's important to create excitement in your diet. Eating a variety of healthy foods will make sure you get all the nutrients you need. Try challenging yourself to taste a new fruit or vegetable every week. It's a fun (and healthy) strategy!

2. Hydration: Lubricating the Core

Hydration is like the grease lubricating a machine, ensuring its parts are well-oiled. It assists in maintaining muscle flexibility, facilitates digestion, and helps to keep skin glowing, all of which are beneficial to the effectiveness of our core movements. The common advice is to drink a minimum of eight glasses of water a day, but don't forget to listen to your body and make adjustments on days when you're more active, and in hot weather.

- Pro Tip: You can put slices of cucumber or lemon in the water for a more appealing taste. These create tasty and refreshing flavors and provide a small vitamin boost.

3. Mindful Eating: Syncing Mind and Body

Mindfulness is a concept that has been incorporated into our workout sessions, including the practices presented in Chapter Seven. Here are some tips to incorporate these principles into your eating habits. Pay attention to your food, or as I like to call it, practice mindful eating. Don't distract yourselves with television or social media while eating, and pay attention to the quality of the foods you consume. This practice assists digestion and allows the identification of satiety signals, reducing the risk of overeating.

Activity: The 'first bite' exercise is recommended. Try for a moment to recall how it feels to eat the first piece of food—make sure to shut your eyes and focus on the taste and the smell. It's a great way to be aware of what you're eating and experience the food you eat.

4. Portion Control: Small Servings for a Strong Core

Aging is characterized by a progressive reduction in the basal metabolic rate due to a decline in energy requirements. That's why portion control is even more critical now than at other times of life, because it's easier to gain weight when consuming high-energy foods and drinks, overloading the body with calories. Try using small plates to help you cut down your portion sizes without necessarily feeling like it's a forced decision.

- Remember: Avoid eating large portions, even at meals. It's generally healthier to have several small meals a day than more traditional large ones.

5. Strategic Snacking: Energy for Core Stability

As you may recall from our exercise snacks in Chapter 8, it's helpful to think of your daily snacks as mini-fuel stops for your body. Choose to eat high-fiber, high-protein snacks such as Greek yogurt, a small bowl of nuts, or an apple with natural peanut butter. These foods have low glycemic indexes, which allows them to keep you feeling full for a longer time and supply you with the energy required for your exercise routines.

Snack Idea: At the beginning of each week, prepare a batch of trail mix consisting of nuts, seeds, and a small serving of dried fruits to have during snack time.

6. Varied Diet: A Spectrum of Nutrients

We've all heard the adage, 'variety is the spice of life.' Well, I think we can also say something akin to 'variety is the nutrient of life'. It's important to consume various kinds of foods to obtain all the nutrients you need for optimal health and core strength. They're vital for your health and to get the most out of the exercises we've talked about in this book. Maintain a balanced diet plan that includes proteins, carbohydrates, fats, vitamins, and minerals to avoid missing out on any nutrients.

Challenge: Take turns planning a 'colorful meal' once a week, with each dish containing as many colors as you can find. This means including plenty of vegetables. This is one way to ensure that you get a lot of nutrients from different foods, and it makes your meal visually appealing.

7. The Pleasure Principle: Enjoying What You Eat

Food is one of life's greatest pleasures, and you deserve to enjoy your meals. As we mentioned in Chapter 9, it's important to enjoy the journey, whether it is moving your body or eating healthy food.

Moderation is key. It's okay to indulge in unhealthy but delicious foods sometimes, but just have small amounts. For example, if you love cake or ice cream, just have a little bit as special treats. As long as you maintain a healthy diet overall, there's no need to feel guilty.

- Tip: Mindfully savor your desserts. Take a slower pace when eating them to fully enjoy each mouthful. This will not only make the act of eating more fulfilling but also make you less likely to eat too much.

Closing: Nourishing for Longevity

I wrote this chapter as not merely a guide to proper nutrition, but also as an exploration of how to enjoy and view food as fuel and a source of delight. By making the effort to eat a healthy and varied diet just like we vary and optimize the exercises in our fitness regimen, we will be healthier, stronger, and more focused on all other aspects of our lives. Here's to savoring every bite and spoonful, and embracing every moment because that feeds the soul. Here's to great health, hearty chuckles, and bellies filled with vibrant and tasty dishes that fuel our centers, and our joy!

Conclusion

So, it's time to say goodbye! Thank you for following me through the last few pages of this adventure. Can you believe it? Like me, you probably feel a combination of pride, enthusiasm, and that tinge of emotion when a good book comes to a close. But before we bid this chapter of our lives goodbye, let's celebrate, dance, and look forward to the next chapters we'll face with renewed spirit and knowledge.

The Road We've Traveled

I bet you remember the moment when you first chose to read this book. It could be that you wanted a change or were interested in how you could improve your health and well-being in these wonderful years. Regardless of what you had in mind at the start, look at you now – you're not only a reader but an active one. You've taken up new tasks, discovered how to feed your body and spirit, and toned up your muscles and character.

Celebrating the Victories, Big and Small

There is one thing that I'd most like you to remember from all the things I've talked about – the need to rejoice at every achievement, no matter how small it may seem. Did you warm up before the exercise? Perhaps you cooked some new vegetable dish from Chapter 10 that you enjoyed eating? Celebrate it all! These are the triumphs in our health and fitness journey. They're like signposts of the journey so far.

It's important to remember that there are always some failures, but they are crucial components of the journey. Perhaps there were days when just getting out of bed was a task, or there were moments when the idea of devouring another salad was the last thing you wanted to do. It's all a process of growth and change. This challenge is a blessing, a chance to learn, evolve, adapt, and continue with more knowledge and motivation.

The Wisdom We've Gained

Before we conclude this chapter, let's consider what you've learned. Apart from the workouts and eating plans, you've gained the ability to hear and understand your body. You've learned how to challenge yourself, yet not cross the line, and how to fuel yourself with food, love, and tolerance.

We've also unlocked the most fundamental secret to maintaining our health and happiness: joy. Yes, joy! The beauty of this transformation is that delight has been found in everyday actions, walks, eating, and breaks. It's not just about living longer but living better, living each day to the fullest without compromising our health.

Looking Ahead with Heart and Hope

So, what comes next? Well, that's the fun part – it's your turn to write the story from now on. You now have this book's exercises and recipes, as well as the confidence in yourself that you can achieve whatever you desire. Perhaps you'll go back to some chapters to improve on certain techniques, or even try out new ones that further challenge your core and spirit.

Therefore, keep on setting goals, keep on discovering, and keep on seeking new opportunities and experiences. And, most importantly, keep smiling! Yes, even if you stumble during the balance pose. But who needs crunches when you can exercise your abs with laughter?

A Toast to You, My Friend

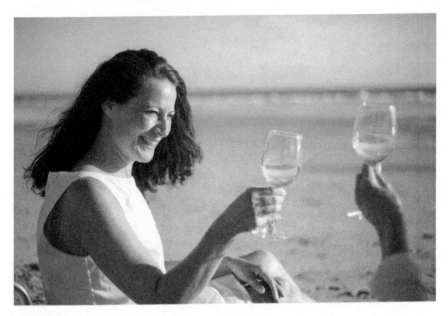

So, before we go our separate ways, let me take a moment to pretend that we're both toasting to your health with a glass of something. This is to the early morning stretches, the home-cooked meals when fast food was more appealing, the push for one more exercise attempt, and the time spent recuperating.

You understand now that one is never too old to live life to the fullest, to build up not only muscle but also passion for life. I'm grateful you let me be a part of your journey. So, let the beats of your heart guide you through these wonderful years with elegance, power, and happiness.

Until we see each other again, be bright, be great, and always know there is tomorrow. Here is to you, here is to your health, and here is to all the ways we can live our lives to the fullest, at any age. Cheers!

Resources

CHAPTER ONE

Kumar, P., & Saini, P. (2023). Effect of kinesio taping in acute low back pain. ResearchGate.

Kao, S. L., Hsiao, M. L., Wang, J. H., & Chen, C. S. (2024). Effects of integrated intrinsic foot muscle exercise with foot core training device on balance and body composition among community-dwelling adults aged 60 and older. BMC Geriatrics.

Li, M., Tian, Y., Wang, C., & Wang, J. (2024). Study on the Independent and Joint Effects of Physical Activity and Sleep on Low Back Pain in Middle-aged and Elderly Adults. Chinese General Practice.

Qi, B., Wang, Z., Cao, Y., & Zhao, H. (2024). Study on the treatment of osteoarthritis by acupuncture combined with traditional Chinese medicine based on pathophysiological mechanism: A review. Medicine.

Dawande, R., Panda, M., Fahim, T., & Kshirsagar, A. (2024). Impact of Russian Current Combined With Close and Open Kinetic Chain Strengthening Exercises on ACL Revision Reconstruction Using Allograft-A Case Report. Kinésithérapie, la Revue.

Chen, E. H., Presta, D., & Bergdahl, A. (2024). Five Weeks of Online Blood Flow Restricted Resistance Training on Postural Stability of Older Adults. International Journal of Exercise Science.

Sullivan, G. M., Pomidor, A. K., & Brummel-Smith, K. (2024). Motivational Interviewing for Older Adults. In Exercise for Aging Adults: A Guide for Practitioners.

Gupta, R., Quintana, J. O., Reddy, N., & Ayotte, S. (2024). A National 20-year Analysis of Weight Lifting–related Injuries and Fractures Among Adolescents. Journal of Pediatric Orthopaedics.

Xu, W., Zhao, X., Zeng, M., Wu, S., He, Y., & Zhou, M. (2024). Exercise for frailty research frontiers: a bibliometric analysis and systematic review. Frontiers in Medicine.

Koch Esteves, N. A. (2024). Regional blood flow in the human leg with local heating and low-intensity exercise in young and old humans. Brunel University Research Archive.

Recenti, F., Dell'Isola, A., Giardulli, B., & Testa, M. (2024). Association between metabolic conditions and satisfaction with care in people with knee or hip osteoarthritis: a survey-based study. Osteoarthritis and Cartilage.

Maru, M., & Tomioka, A. (2024). Who and What Did We Miss in Childhood Cancer Survivor Research? Cancer Nursing.

Camanho, L., & Carneiro, J. (2024). Armando de Almeida. A Lesson in Resistance in Portuguese Running Culture. Vista: Revista de Cultural Visual.

Ukachukwu, A. E. K., Adeolu, A. A., Adeleye, A. O., & others. (2024). Neurosurgical practice, training, and research capacity assessment in Nigeria: A methodological approach. World Neurosurgery.

Gzik, M., Paszenda, Z., Piętka, E., Tkacz, E., & Milewski, K. (2024). Innovations in Biomedical Engineering 2023. Springer.

CHAPTER TWO

Hemmatizad, F., RafeiBoroujeni, M., & Salehi, H. (2023). The Effect of Task Complexity on Bilateral Transfer in Older Adults. Journals at the University of Tehran. Retrieved from

Huyghe, E., Ducrot, Q., Kassab, D., Faix, A., & Hupertan, V. (2024). Survey on vasectomy practices in France in 2022. ResearchGate.

Manifield, J., Alexiou, C., Megaritis, D., & Baker, K. (2024). Effects of inspiratory muscle training on thoracoabdominal volume regulation in older adults: a randomised controlled trial. Respiratory Physiology & Neurobiology.

Ryan, J. M., Simiceva, A., Toale, C., & Eppich, W. (2024). Assessing current handover practices in surgery: A survey of non-consultant hospital doctors in Ireland. The Surgeon. R

Singh, K. J. (2024). Mycelex-g. Retrieved from https://www.fbs.edu.pl/docs1/order-mycelex-g-no-rx/

Cassemiliano, G., Farche, A. C. S., & others. (2024). Physical Capacity and Its Relationship With Depressive Symptoms, Quality of Life and Sedentary Behavior in Community-Dwelling Older Adults: A Longitudinal Study. Journal of Aging and Physical Activity.

Carraro, U. (2024). Personalized Full-Body In-Bed Gym at home: lessons from personal experiences. Mental Wellness.

Chan, Y. L. E., Lin, W. S., Lai, H. C., Hung, C. Y., & others. (2024). Changes in cognitive function after a 12-week POWER rehabilitation in older adults with schizophrenia and frailty. Asia-Pacific Psychiatry. Retrieved from

Bianchi, D., Sethi, N. K., Velasco, G., & others. (2024). Care of The Older Fighter: Position Statement of the Association of Ringside Physicians. The Physician and Sportsmedicine.

Chen, G., Yu, D., Wang, Y., Ma, Z., Bi, M., Lu, L., & others. (2024). Effects of Preoperative Combined with Postoperative Progressive Resistance Training on Muscle Strength, Gait, Balance and Function in Patients Undergoing Total Hip Arthroplasty. Clinical Interventions in Aging.

Sousa, C. V., Hoyos, P., Buesgens, D., Villiger, E., Thuany, M., & others. (2024). The Neglected Category of Sub-elite Athletes in Ironman Triathlon: Participation, Performance, and Implications for Fitness Assessment. Research Square.

Rangabprai, Y., Mitranun, W., & Mitarnun, W. (2024). Effect of 60-min Single Bout of Resistance Exercise, Reformer Pilates, on Vascular Function Parameters in Older Adults: A Randomized Crossover Study. Gerontology. Retrieved from

Desmond, A. (2024). British Aborigines. Open Book Publishers.

Ren, K. (2024). Building Learning Power (BLP) to Senior High School Students Towards Enhanced Learning Program. Journal of Education and Educational Research.

Lin, K. K. Y., Huang, C. W., Chen, S. H., Lee, J. J., & others. (2024). Rehabilitation Program for Post-Laryngectomy Patients Following Ileocolon Flap Transfer for Voice Reconstruction--An essential part of success.

CHAPTER THREE

Das, T., & Bandyopadhyay, N. (2023). Pilates Exercises, Types, and Its Importance: An Overview.

Zwakhalen, S. M. G., Cremer, S., & others. (2023). The AOL Nursing Guideline.

Uddin, M. R. (2024). Sociodemographic, Clinical & Biochemical Features in Children with Nephrotic Syndrome: A Study in a Tertiary Care Hospital of Bangladesh.

Nagai, T., Miyagami, M., Nakamura, S., Sakamoto, K., & others. (2024). Relationship between sacral-abdominal wall distance, movement performance, and spinal alignment in osteoporosis: a retrospective study.

Tryfonos, C., Chrysafi, M., Papadopoulou, S. K., & others. (2024). Life and physical activity, sociodemographic and anthropometric parameters, and serum biomarkers in community-dwelling older adults with multiple sclerosis.

Yin, L., Wang, C., Zhao, W., Yang, X., Guo, Y., Mu, D., & others. (2024). Association between muscular tissue desaturation and acute kidney injury in older patients undergoing major abdominal surgery: a prospective cohort study.

Kokoszyński, D., Żochowska-Kujawska, J., Kotowicz, M., & others. (2024). Carcass characteristics, physicochemical traits, texture and microstructure of young and spent quails meat.

Xu, W., Zhao, X., Zeng, M., Wu, S., He, Y., Zhou, M. (2024). Exercise for frailty research frontiers: a bibliometric analysis and systematic review.

Fukushima, N., Masuda, T., Tsuboi, K., Yuda, M., & others. (2024). Prognostic significance of preoperative osteosarcopenia on patient outcomes after emergency surgery for gastrointestinal perforation.

Ganjeh Amineh, M., Mohammadi, B., Rabiei, M., & others. (2024). The effect of eight weeks core stability training on improving the physical performance in parkour athletes Male 12 to 20 years old (semi-experimental study).

Chen, E. H., Presta, D., Bergdahl, A., & others. (2024). Five Weeks of Online Blood Flow Restricted Resistance Training on Postural Stability of Older Adults. Retrieved from

Samaei, S., Pincu, Y. (2024). Associations between walking parameters and health outcomes in older adults with metabolic syndrome.

CHAPTER FOUR

Hsu, F.-Y., Tsai, K.-L., Lee, C.-L., Chang, W.-D., & Chang, N. (2020). Effects of Dynamic Stretching Combined With Static Stretching, Foam Rolling, or Vibration Rolling as a Warm-Up Exercise on Athletic Performance in Elite Table Tennis Players. Journal of Sport Rehabilitation.

Hernández-Martínez, J., Castillo-Cerda, M., Vera-Assaoka, T., Carter-Truillier, B., Herrera-Valenzuela, T., Guzmán-Muñoz, E., Branco, B., Jofré-Saldía, E., & Valdés-Badilla, P. (2022). Warm-Up and Handgrip Strength in Physically Inactive Chilean Older Females According to Baseline Nutritional Status. International Journal of Environmental Research and Public Health.

Van Raalte, J. V., Brewer, B., Cornelius, A., Keeler, M., & Gudjenov, C. (2019). Effects of a Mental Warmup on the Workout Readiness and Stress of College Student Exercisers. Journal of Functional Morphology and Kinesiology.

Neves, P., Alves, A. R., Marinho, D., & Neiva, H. (2021). Warming-Up for Resistance Training and Muscular Performance: A Narrative Review. Recent Advances in Sport Science.

Ribeiro, B., Pereira, A., Neves, P., Marinho, D., Marques, M., & Neiva, H. (2021). The effect of warm-up in resistance training and strength performance: a systematic review. Motricidade, 17, 87-94.

Vora, M., & Arora, M. (2019). An Analysis of the Evidence Base Relating to the Role of Warm-Up and Stretching in Reduction of Injury Risk in Athletes. Orthopedics and Sports Medicine Open Access Journal.

Myburgh, G. K., Pfeifer, C., & Hecht, C. J. (2020). Warm-ups for Youth Athletes: Making the First 15-Minutes Count. Strength and Conditioning Journal.

Boguszewski, D., Adamczyk, J., Hanc, A., Szymanska, A., Chełchowska, S., & Białoszewski, D. (2021). Classic sports massage vs. Chinese self-massage. Which one is more effective in warm-up? Biomedical Human Kinetics, 13, 97-102.

Kaufmann, J.-E., Nelissen, R., Stubbe, J., & Gademan, M. (2022). Neuromuscular Warm-Up is Associated with Fewer Overuse Injuries in Ballet Dancers Compared to Traditional Ballet-Specific Warm-Up. Journal of Dance Medicine Science, 26, 244-254.

Chen, C.-H., Hsu, C.-H., Chu, L., Chiu, C.-H., Yang, W., Yu, K.-W., & Ye, X. (2022). Acute Effects of Static Stretching Combined with Vibration and Nonvibration Foam Rolling on the Cardiovascular Responses and Functional Fitness of Older Women with Prehypertension. Biology, 11.

CHAPTER FIVE

Nie, Q., & Rogers, W. (2019). Understanding needs and challenges of health self-management activities for older adults with mobility limitations. Innovation in Aging, 3, S352-S353.

Atoyebi, O., Labbé, D., Prescott, M., Mahmood, A., Routhier, F., Miller, W., & Mortenson, W. (2019). Mobility challenges among older adult mobility device users. Current Geriatrics Reports, 1-9.

Koon, L., Remillard, E. T., Mitzner, T., & Rogers, W. (2020). Aging concerns, challenges, and everyday solution strategies (ACCESS) for adults aging with a long-term mobility disability. Disability and Health Journal, 13, 100936.

Remillard, E. T., Fausset, C., & Fain, W. (2019). Aging with long-term mobility impairment: Maintaining activities of daily living via selection, optimization, and compensation. The Gerontologist, 59(3), 559-569.

Nie, Q., Koon, L., Khamzina, M., & Rogers, W. (2020). Understanding exercise challenges and barriers for older adults with mobility disabilities. Proceedings of the Human Factors and Ergonomics Society Annual Meeting, 64, 1297-1301.

McKay, M. A., Cohn, A., & O'Connor, M. (2023). The symptom experience of older adults with mobility difficulties: Qualitative interviews. Journal of Applied Gerontology.

Billot, M., Calvani, R., Urtamo, A., Sánchez-Sánchez, J., Ciccolari-Micaldi, C., Chang, M., ... & Freiberger, E. (2020). Preserving mobility in older adults with physical frailty and sarcopenia: Opportunities, challenges, and recommendations for physical activity interventions. Clinical Interventions in Aging, 15, 1675-1690.

Ramadhani, W., & Rogers, W. A. (2022). Understanding home activity challenges of older adults aging with long-term mobility disabilities: Recommendations for home environment design. Journal of Aging and Environment, 37, 341-363.

Anton, S., Cruz-Almeida, Y., Singh, A., Alpert, J., Bensadon, B., Cabrera, M., ... & Pahor, M. (2020). Innovations in geroscience to enhance mobility in older adults. Experimental Gerontology, 142, 111123.

Resna, R., Lazuardi, L., Werdati, S., & Rochmah, W. (2019). Development of detection instrument models for mobility impairment in the older adults based on a mobile health nursing application in a public health center. Jurnal Ners, 14(3), 86-92.

CHAPTER SIX

Oliveira, M. R., Fabrin, L. F., Gil, A. W. O., Benassi, G., Camargo, M. Z., & da Silva, R. A. (2021). Acute effect of core stability and sensory-motor exercises on postural control during sitting and standing positions in young adults. Journal of Bodywork and Movement Therapies, 28, 98-103.

Kemeny, B., Bright, H., Digman, L., McCormack, K., Page, R., & Setto, M. (2023). Is education enough? Seated yoga and falls prevention for older adults. Innovation in Aging, 7, 1169-1170.

Nikhade, N., & Phalke, V. (2023). Effect of chair Suryanamaskar with strength training on functional fitness in frail older adults: A research protocol for a randomized controlled trial. Journal of Clinical and Diagnostic Research.

Xu, Y. (2022). Impact of core fitness on balance performance in the elderly. Revista Brasileira de Medicina do Esporte.

Lim, S., Meredith, S., Agnew, S., Clift, E., Ibrahim, K., & Roberts, H. (2023). Volunteer-led online group exercise for older adults: A feasibility and acceptability study. Age and Ageing.

Ponde, K., Agrawal, R., & Chikte, N. K. (2021). Effect of core stabilization exercises on balance performance in older adults. International Journal of Contemporary Medicine.

Wheeler, M. J., Dunstan, D., Smith, B., Smith, K. J., Scheer, A., Lewis, J., Naylor, L., Heinonen, I., Ellis, K., Cerin, E., Ainslie, P., & Green, D. (2019). Morning exercise mitigates the impact of prolonged sitting on cerebral blood flow in older adults. Journal of Applied Physiology, 126(4), 1049-1055.

Coyle, P. C., Perera, S., Albert, S., Freburger, J., VanSwearingen, J., & Brach, J. (2020). Potential long-term impact of "On The Move" group-exercise program on falls and healthcare utilization in older adults: An exploratory analysis of a randomized controlled trial. BMC Geriatrics, 20.

Bai, X., Soh, K., Dev Omar Dev, R., Talib, O., Xiao, W., Soh, K. L., Ong, S. L., Zhao, C., Galeru, O., & Casaru, C. (2022). Aerobic exercise combination intervention to improve physical performance among the elderly: A systematic review. Frontiers in Physiology, 12.

Veneri, D., & Gannotti, M. (2021). Take a seat for yoga with seniors: A scoping review. OBM Geriatrics.

CHAPTER SEVEN

Tollár, J., Nagy, F., Moizs, M., Tóth, B. E., Sanders, L., & Hortobágyi, T. (2019). Diverse Exercises Similarly Reduce Older Adults' Mobility Limitations. Medicine & Science in Sports & Exercise.

Xu, Y. (2022). Impact of Core Fitness on Balance Performance in the Elderly. Revista Brasileira de Medicina do Esporte.

Alqahtani, B., Sparto, P., Whitney, S., Greenspan, S., Perera, S., VanSwearingen, J., & Brach, J. (2019). Effect of Community-Based Group Exercise Interventions on Standing Balance and Strength in Independent Living Older Adults. Journal of Geriatric Physical Therapy.

Bai, X., Soh, K., Dev Omar Dev, R., Talib, O., Xiao, W., Soh, K. L., Ong, S. L., Zhao, C., Galeru, O., & Casaru, C. (2022). Aerobic Exercise Combination Intervention to Improve Physical Performance Among the Elderly: A Systematic Review. Frontiers in Physiology.

Lai, Z., Pang, H., Hu, X., Dong, K., & Wang, L. (2021). Effects of Intrinsic-Foot-Muscle Exercise Combined with Lower Extremity Resistance Training on Postural Stability in Older Adults with Fall Risk: Study Protocol for a Randomised Controlled Trial. Trials.

Oliveira, M. R., Fabrin, L. F., Gil, A. W. O., Benassi, G., Camargo, M. Z., & da Silva, R. A. (2021). Acute Effect of Core Stability and Sensory-Motor Exercises on Postural Control During Sitting and Standing Positions in Young Adults. Journal of Bodywork and Movement Therapies.

Tosi, F. C., Lin, S. M., Gomes, G., Aprahamian, I., Nakagawa, N. K., Viveiro, L., Bacha, J. R., Jacob-Filho, W., & Pompéu, J. (2021). A Multidimensional Program Including Standing Exercises, Health Education, and Telephone Support to Reduce Sedentary Behavior in Frail Older Adults: Randomized Clinical Trial. Experimental Gerontology.

Salsabila, B. I., Rahman, F., & Lindoyo, Y. (2023). Different Effects of Single-Leg Stance Exercise and Bridging Exercise with Core Stability Exercise on Older Adults' Balance. Exercise Science.

Zhang, W., Liu, X., Liu, H., Zhang, X., Song, T., Gao, B., Ding, D., Li, H., & Yan, Z. (2023). Effects of Aerobic and Combined Aerobic-Resistance Exercise on Motor Function in Sedentary Older Adults: A Clinical Trial. Journal of Back and Musculoskeletal Rehabilitation.

Fang, Q., Ghanouni, P., Anderson, S., Touchett, H., Shirley, R., Fang, F., & Fang, C. (2019). Effects of Exergaming on Balance of Healthy Older Adults: A Systematic Review and Meta-Analysis of Randomized Controlled Trials. Games for Health Journal.

CHAPTER EIGHT

Wheeler, M. J., Dunstan, D., Smith, B., Smith, K. J., Scheer, A., Lewis, J., Naylor, L., Heinonen, I., Ellis, K., Cerin, E., Ainslie, P., & Green, D. (2019). Morning exercise mitigates the impact of prolonged sitting on cerebral blood flow in older adults. Journal of Applied Physiology, 126(4), 1049-1055.

Park, J., & Kim, J. (2023). Effects of cooling glove on the human body's recovery after exercise and improvement of exercise ability. Technology and Health Care, 31, 259-269.

Winett, R., & Ogletree, A. (2019). Evidence-based, high-intensity exercise and physical activity for compressing morbidity in older adults: A narrative review. Innovation in Aging, 3.

Tollár, J., Nagy, F., Moizs, M., Tóth, B. E., Sanders, L., & Hortobágyi, T. (2019). Diverse exercises similarly reduce older adults' mobility limitations. Medicine & Science in Sports & Exercise.

Sadacharan, C. (2022). Effects of multi-component exercise on older adults with chronic conditions. The Journal of Sports Medicine and Physical Fitness.

Marriott, C. F. S., Petrella, A., Marriott, E., Boa Sorte Silva, N. C., & Petrella, R. (2021). High-intensity interval training in older adults: A scoping review. Sports Medicine - Open, 7, 1-24.

Seol, J., Fujii, Y., Inoue, T., Kitano, N., Tsunoda, K., & Okura, T. (2020). Effects of morning versus evening home-based exercise on subjective and objective sleep parameters in older adults: A randomized controlled trial. Journal of Geriatric Psychiatry and Neurology, 34, 232-242.

Větrovský, T., Omcirk, D., Maleček, J., Stastny, P., Šteffl, M., & Tufano, J. (2021). Morning fatigue and structured exercise interact to affect non-exercise physical activity of fit and healthy older adults. BMC Geriatrics, 21.

Frost, N., Weinborn, M., Gignac, G. E., Rainey-Smith, S., Markovic, S., Gordon, N., Sohrabi, H., Laws, S., Martins, R., Peiffer, J., & Brown, B. (2020). A randomized controlled trial of high-intensity exercise and executive functioning in cognitively normal older adults. The American Journal of Geriatric Psychiatry, 28(12), 1330-1340.

Seol, J., Park, I., Kokudo, C., Zhang, S., Suzuki, C., Yajima, K., Satoh, M., Tokuyama, K., & Okura, T. (2020). Distinct effects of low-intensity physical activity in the evening on sleep quality in older women: A comparison of exercise and housework. Experimental Gerontology, 143, 111165.

CHAPTER NINE

Teixeira, C. V., Evangelista, A., Marta dos Santos Silva, M., Bocalini, D., Silva-Grigoletto, M., & Behm, D. G. (2019). Ten Important Facts About Core Training. ACSM'S Health & Fitness Journal.

Luo, S., Soh, K., Soh, K. L., Sun, H., Nasiruddin, N. J. M., Du, C., & Zhai, X. (2021). Effect of Core Training on Skill Performance Among Athletes: A Systematic Review. Frontiers in Physiology.

Pawlina, M., Ziętara, K., Raksa, K., Nowakowska, K., & Lewkowicz, M. (2022). Maximizing the efficiency of resistance training. Journal of Education, Health and Sport.

Wang, T., Liu, Y.-X., & Weng, Z. (2022). CORE STRENGTH TRAINING IN UNIVERSITY FEMALE TENNIS PLAYERS. Revista Brasileira de Medicina do Esporte.

Doğanay, M., Bingül, B. M., & Álvarez-García, C. (2020). Effect of core training on speed, quickness, and agility in young male football players. The Journal of Sports Medicine and Physical Fitness.

Duchateau, J., Stragier, S., Baudry, S., & Carpentier, A. (2020). Strength Training: in Search of Optimal Strategies to Maximize Neuromuscular Performance. Exercise and Sport Sciences Reviews.

Lupowitz, L. G. (2023). Comprehensive Approach to Core Training in Sports Physical Therapy: Optimizing Performance and Minimizing Injuries. International Journal of Sports Physical Therapy.

Dong, K., Yu, T., & Chun, B. (2023). Effects of Core Training on Sport-Specific Performance of Athletes: A Meta-Analysis of Randomized Controlled Trials. Behavioral Sciences.

Sasaki, S., Tsuda, E., Yamamoto, Y., Maeda, S., Kimura, Y., Fujita, Y., & Ishibashi, Y. (2019). Core-Muscle Training and Neuromuscular Control of Lower Limb and Trunk. Journal of Athletic Training.

Karpiński, J., Rejdych, W., Brzozowska, D., Gołaś, A., Sadowski, W., Swinarew, A., Stachura, A., Gupta, S., & Stanula, A. (2019). The effects of a 6-week core exercises on swimming performance of national level swimmers. PLoS ONE.

CHAPTER TEN

Fritzen, A., Lundsgaard, A. M., & Kiens, B. (2019). Dietary Fuels in Athletic Performance. Annual Review of Nutrition.

Mardiana, M., Kartini, A., Sutiningsih, D., Suroto, S., & Muhtar, M. S. (2023). Literature Review: Nutrition Supplementation for Muscle Fatigue in Athletes. Jurnal Keolahragaan.

Papadopoulou, S. (2020). Rehabilitation Nutrition for Injury Recovery of Athletes: The Role of Macronutrient Intake. Nutrients.

Kim, J., & Kim, E.-K. (2020). Nutritional Strategies to Optimize Performance and Recovery in Rowing Athletes. Nutrients.

Nielsen, L. L. K., Lambert, M. N. T., & Jeppesen, P. B. (2020). The Effect of Ingesting Carbohydrate and Proteins on Athletic Performance: A Systematic Review and Meta-Analysis of Randomized Controlled Trials. Nutrients.

Braun-Trocchio, R., Graybeal, A., Kreutzer, A., Warfield, E., Renteria, J., Harrison, K., Williams, A., & Moss, K. (2022). Recovery Strategies in Endurance Athletes. Journal of Functional Morphology and Kinesiology.

Russo, I., Della Gatta, P. D., Garnham, A., Porter, J., Burke, L., & Costa, R. (2021). The Effects of an Acute "Train-Low" Nutritional Protocol on Markers of Recovery Optimization in Endurance-Trained Male Athletes. International Journal of Sports Physiology and Performance.

Larsen, M. S., Clausen, D., Jørgensen, A. A., Mikkelsen, U. R., & Hansen, M. (2019). Presleep Protein Supplementation Does Not Improve Recovery During Consecutive Days of Intense Endurance Training: A Randomized Controlled Trial. International Journal of Sport Nutrition and Exercise Metabolism.

Arroyo-Cerezo, A., Cerrillo, I., Ortega, Á., & Fernández-Pachón, M. (2021). Intake of Branched Chain Amino Acids Favors Post-Exercise Muscle Recovery and May Improve Muscle Function: Optimal Dosage Regimens and Consumption Conditions. The Journal of Sports Medicine and Physical Fitness.

O'Connor, E., Mündel, T., & Barnes, M. (2022). Nutritional Compounds to Improve Post-Exercise Recovery. Nutrients.

Printed in Great Britain
by Amazon

57381104R00089